A Quest for Certainty

Essays on Health Care
Economics, 1930-1970

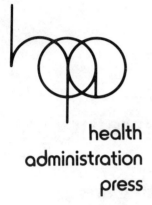

A Quest

for Certainty

Essays on Health Care
Economics, 1930-1970

C. Rufus Rorem, Ph.D., C.P.A.

Health Administration Press
Ann Arbor, Michigan
1982

Library of Congress Cataloging in Publication Data

Rorem, C. Rufus (Clarence Rufus), 1894-
  A quest for certainty

  Bibliography: p.
  1. Medical economics—United States—Addresses,
essays, lectures.   2. Medical care—United States—
Addresses, essays, lectures.   I. Title. [DNLM: 1. In-
surance, Health.   2. Health planning.   3. Health services
—Economics, W 74 R787q]
  RA410.53.R66   338.4'3368382'00973   81-20076
  ISBN 0-914904-75-2   AACR2

Health Administration Press
School of Public Health
The University of Michigan
Ann Arbor, Michigan 48109
313-764-1380

Contents

Foreword: Prospect for Health   *vii*

Comment by Walter J. McNerney   *xi*

Acknowledgments   *xv*

Part One: Health Care as Public Service

Comment by Victor R. Fuchs   *3*

Capital Investment and the Public (1930)   *6*

Private Group Clinics (1931)   *13*

Some Economic Issues in Hospital Management (1932)   *19*

The Hospital as a Medical Service Center (1932)   *28*

Inseparable Team: Physician and Hospital (1950)   *35*

Patterns and Problems of Group Medical Practice (1950)   *39*

Need Every Hospital Offer an Obstetric Service? (1966)   *50*

Part Two: Group Payment for Health Care

Comment by Robert M. Sigmond   *59*

Sickness Insurance in the United States (1932)   *62*

Group Hospitalization: Mecca or Mirage? (1933)   *72*

A Model Plan for Group Hospitalization (1934)   *83*

Health Insurance: Rorem vs. Fishbein (1939)   *89*

The Blue Cross Story: U.S. Senate Hearings (1946)   *99*

Health Service in England (It Could Happen
   Here) (1947)   *109*

Commercial Insurance (1953)   *114*

Part Three: Health Care Finance and Planning

Comment by Herbert E. Klarman   *121*

Fixed Charges in Hospital Accounting (1931)   *125*

Why Hospital Costs Have Risen (1950)   *131*

Standards and Priorities for Areawide Planning (1954)   *138*

Hospital Pricing: Theory and Practice (1958)   *149*

The Hospital of 1986 (1961)   *158*

Areawide Planning Is Here to Stay (1964)   *163*

Changing Capital Needs and Financing (1968)   *169*

The Economics of Geriatric Health Care (1970)   *174*

Afterword: The Continuing Uncertainty   *183*

Appendix A: Chronological List of Books and Brochures by
    C. Rufus Rorem (1928–1970)   *188*

Appendix B: Articles by C. Rufus Rorem Published in Journals and
    Magazines (1925–1971)   *190*

Foreword: Prospect for Health

During the year 1927, a national Committee on the Costs of Medical Care (CCMC) began a five-year study of the provision and financing of health services for the American people. It was a time of full employment, high wages, and moderate prices for goods and services, including health care. But there was widespread criticism of prices for health services, and a general belief that the benefits of medical knowledge and skill were not readily available to the average person. Six philanthropic foundations contributed a total of about one million dollars to support the project. Two others refused to help, on the grounds that research was unnecessary and the time had come for action.

I served as a staff economist for the CCMC, and helped to prepare its final report, which was published in October of 1932. I devoted full time until January 1966 to the study and development of health care finance and administration—at the national level in Chicago, and also in Philadelphia, Pittsburgh, and New York City.

CCMC studies revealed that total health care expenditures for the year 1929 were equal to about four percent of the Gross National Product. Ninety percent of the capital investment in hospitals and professional personnel had been provided through taxation and philanthropy. These proportions seemed reasonable for an enlightened nation. Health may properly be regarded as wealth. Unattended sickness or disability is a waste of community resources, therefore a menace to public safety and convenience. Access to existing health services is a basic right, essential to the effective pursuit of happiness.

The CCMC documented the fact that statistics of national totals and averages were of little comfort to individuals and families in their search for health care. No one could tell when he would be sick or disabled, or how much his health care would cost. Some people would receive no service during a year. Others might face expenditures of several thousand dollars, even more than one's total annual income or life savings. It was not the cost, it was the uncertainty that gave rise to complaints about the costs and availability of health care.

Health care is fraught with uncertainty for everyone. Various methods have been developed to avoid or reduce the risk. Actual and potential patients have used the devices of insurance and taxation by which health care is placed in the family or community budget along with other necessities. Professionals and institutions have organized groups for medical practice in which specialized knowledge and resources are coordinated to improve quality and reduce costs. Communities have established areawide planning agencies to study, evaluate, and coordinate total facilities and services. Basically all health care activities, including experiments in organization and financing, are components of a comprehensive and continuous *quest for certainty*.

Health care economics deals with effective use of professional personnel and facilities and equitable methods of financing services. It is not directly concerned with medical education, technical skill, scientific advances, or environmental control. The quality of medical care is, of course, affected by general progress in the art and science of medicine. But for an individual patient the value of health care is measured by its availability when needed. Help from a friendly neighbor present at the bedside is more valuable than the professional knowledge of a renowned specialist at the country club. A practitioner's advice must be followed to be effective. A doctor cannot compel a patient to take proper care of himself between office visits.

Health care is an economic commodity, in the sense that the costs of production and consumption can be, and are, measured in terms of money. But health care differs sharply from other commodities. Buyers and sellers do not deal on equal terms in their knowledge about health care. A patient cannot really "beware" in his own interest. No one knows when he will be sick or disabled, or what the experience will cost him. His needs are compulsory, and care cannot always be deferred to a convenient time.

Health care is uniquely personal. A distraught parent cannot suffer pain for a sick child. A busy executive cannot send out for an eye test or chest examination. The need for health care is not adjusted to a patient's resources or annual income. Nor can unsatisfactory service be returned for credit or exchange.

Many studies have demonstrated that health services are most effective when both providers and consumers are least motivated by economic considerations. This means that a practitioner or institution should be free to perform or refuse a service according to a patient's needs, rather than his ability or willingness to pay.

Health care should be businesslike, but I am disturbed when hospital spokesmen and physicians describe their activities as an "industry." In my opinion health care is a broad public service, not private property to be traded over the counter and withheld from those unable or unwilling to pay. Group practice and group payment are effective devices for bringing health care to those who need it. But they were not developed merely to insure survival and adequate income for providers.

No official payment agency can regulate the quality of health care. This must be done by the providers of services and commodities. The paying organizations do not need to influence the quality of medical care directly. But they should use their buying power to negotiate the best possible deals for patients. This includes adequate reimbursement of the personnel and institutions which provide health care.

The early writings selected for this volume were not history when they were published. They described current efforts to achieve certainty in the costs and quality of health care, especially through group practice, group payment, and areawide planning. They correctly anticipated many future developments and included some false prophecies as well. They are reprinted without revision, except for some deletions to avoid repetition and some italics to provide emphasis.

C. RUFUS ROREM
September 1981

Comment

During the celebration of the fiftieth anniversary of the Blue Cross and Blue Shield organizations in 1979, Rufus Rorem conducted a seminar for selected junior executive staff of the American Hospital Association and the Blue Cross and Blue Shield Associations. Galluses, belt, and all, the epitome of certainty, this person, who published his first article in 1927, made a profound impression. The rest of us, in his shadow, were encouraged to see that simply stated reason still has an audience among the younger generation. Still deeply community-oriented and sincere, Rorem spiced his conversation with humor and good, practical sense.

Rufus' interest in prepayment was sparked by his work on the Committee on the Cost of Medical Care from 1928 to 1932 and reinforced by his membership on the Accounting Committee of the American Hospital Association from 1931 to 1941. Correcting the sad shape of internal financial systems led naturally to the broader subject of financing. His wry sense of humor sparkled early. In 1934, when asked how doctors felt about the advent of voluntary prepayment for hospitals, he replied, "The reaction is split between two groups. Fifty percent oppose it because it will lead to socialized medicine, and fifty percent oppose it because medical services are not included." That same year, in discussing what hospitals really want in reimbursement, he said, "More."

The same blend of logic, mission, and perspective that has always made Rufus personally effective makes the essays reprinted in this volume fresh and informative. His messages remain pertinent, including his frequent references to group prepayment, coordinated practice, one class of care, and areawide planning.

In my own enterprise, the Blue Cross and Blue Shield organizations, Rufus is esteemed by common consent as having been an indispensable force at the beginning. As a consultant to an American Hospital Association task force, he was deeply involved in the development of principles and standards promulgated to guide the destiny of widely emerging local Plans. Such standards as not-for-profit operations, no commissions for the enrollment staff, and the necessity of contracts with participating hospitals bear his imprint. The fledgling field could have gone in several directions, but these and other ideas stuck and gave what became Blue Cross and Blue Shield Plans a sense of unity and common destiny. In the concept of a service contract, Rorem and others saw with clarity the desirability of risk sharing not only among subscribers, but also between the Plans and hospitals. Only now are we coming back to a full appreciation of this concept of a flat rate to hospitals and hospital underwriting.

Between 1933 and 1936, Rufus supplied what was badly needed— active leadership. During this period, he spent innumerable hours helping communities start Plans, and he rallied to the cause all who would follow. He wrote prolifically, so much that Plan officials referred to the deluge of ditto copy that came from him as the "purple menace."

Rufus took on all comers when prepayment was not a popular idea among the professions in the health field. With equal facility he debated concepts of depreciation with hospital administrators and the notion of national health insurance with the AMA's Morris Fishbein. The rapid growth of prepayment made it clear where the public stood.

It should be pointed out that Rufus Rorem, although deeply committed to community need, was not rigidly orthodox in manner or temperament. I. S. Falk, with whom Rufus had many spirited discussions, insisted that group practice was needed to make group prepayment work. Rorem supported both but pragmatically accepted either, separately or in any order. He saw group financing and delivery as means to the end, to the goal, of certainty, or at least predictability, and he was flexible regarding means. This reasonableness around basic issues gave the emerging Plans the breathing room they needed to reflect the unique settings of which they were a part. Today, one might suspect that Rufus rejoices at the challenge of wedding prepayment to the task of vertically and horizontally integrating hospitals, or using innovative ways of reshaping the delivery of care through financing. His standards were right: enough rigor to protect against loss of mission, but without the rigidity which would create sectarianism.

Rufus' title for this book is typically provocative. In a day when we are all talking about cost containment, he chooses to throw down the gauntlet and talk about certainty. With this challenge, he reminds us that although a lot has happened since the thirties (e.g., most persons are now covered by some form of protection), the costs of care still are unpredictable, still fall unevenly on individuals and families, and still are often inversely related to income. The nature of expenses may be different today when more chronic diseases and fewer communicable diseases are involved, but the gnawing doubt of who will be at risk is still there. It is no accident, then, that under consumer choice schemes—

the Federal Employee Program, for example—protection is given high value even when more out-of-pocket contributions are involved.

Rufus Rorem left the grand circus of Chicago and an emerging group of Plan prima donnas to go to Philadelphia. E. A. van Steenwyck, an old friend who had created the Blue Cross symbol, headed the Philadelphia Blue Cross Plan. This afforded Rufus an opportunity to operate locally, where he felt the best decisions ultimately are made—closer to the problems and where differences among hospitals, doctors, carriers, management, labor, government, and others could be more sensitively negotiated. Not many people know that, in the thirties, Rufus was against statewide Blue Cross Plans. He felt that Michigan, for instance, should have developed three or four Plans instead of one. Instinctively he focused on the community rather than the nation, despite his national leadership. Perhaps because of this, Rufus thought at first that the Blue Cross concept had limited application. He saw a 10-million voluntary enrollment as maximum; most other experts at the time predicted an even smaller enrollment, if they appreciated the concept at all. In typically understated style, Rufus recently said, "Blue Cross enrollment has exceeded my expectations."

It is interesting to note that the country is coming to the realization that local efforts in health care are critically important. Nationwide governmental solutions rarely work and involve excessive red tape. In 1946, Rufus urged the government to use the private sector by enrolling public assistance beneficiaries in private prepayment plans. Today we talk of a voucher system for Medicare.

Is this book's historical perspective useful to the early or mid-career reader? Clearly it is, whether one's interest is public policy, private financing, or more technical problems. Furthermore, the book is timely in the issues it addresses. Today, when innovative financing rather than comprehensive national health insurance is being actively debated, there is a need for greater understanding of the relationship of financing to organization, distribution, and accountability in the continuing quest for certainty.

WALTER J. MCNERNEY

Acknowledgments

The publisher gratefully acknowledges the assistance of the Health Service Improvement Fund of Blue Cross/Blue Shield of Greater New York in making this book possible.

Thanks are extended to the following publishers, organizations, and periodicals that granted permission to reprint:
American Economic Security, American Journal of Public Health, Bulletin of the American Hospital Association, Charles C. Thomas, Inc., Hospital Accounting, Hospital Financial Management, Hospitals, Journal of Accountancy, Milbank Memorial Fund, Philadelphia Medicine, Pittsburgh Post-Gazette, Rotarian, the Taylor Society, The Modern Hospital, Trustee, University of Chicago Press.

Part One

Health Care as Public Service

Comment

For more than half a century Rufus Rorem has been engaging our thought and concern through informed, closely reasoned, and (as we now know) prophetic articles on almost every aspect of health care. Readers coming to Rorem for the first time will be astounded at his prescience, his ability to cut to the core of complex issues, and his dedication to the discovery of efficient, equitable solutions to difficult problems. Those who have not known Rorem and benefited from his wise counsel may be surprised to find that many of their bright new ideas were carefully spelled out by him in the thirties and forties.

The papers in this section are devoted to questions concerning the organization of health care. The physician and the hospital—Rorem's "inseparable team"—are the main subject. Questions of finance and reimbursement, while not central in these papers, enter the discussion because of their close relation to organization. Early in his career, Rorem identified major influences affecting health care: the trend toward greater specialization, the increasing importance of capital equipment, and the pervasive influence of uncertainty.* His analysis of these forces led him to the following conclusions:

1. The cost of health care should be borne by the entire population through private insurance and tax-supported government programs. It should not fall only on the ill nor should it be based on a "Robin Hood" approach to the pricing of health services.

2. Attention to the cost of capital is essential if resources are to be allocated efficiently. In particular, unnecessary expansion of hospitals or duplication of facilities must be avoided.

3. The patient (or the public) is interested in the total cost of an illness episode, not in the details of the division between the physician and the hospital. The physician and the hospital, therefore, are to some degree in competition with each other for the health care dollar.

4. The physician is the key person in the health care effort because he influences the entire process of care.

*Cf. Kenneth Arrow, Uncertainty and the welfare economics of medical care, *American Economic Review* 53: 941, 1963.

5. The group practice of medicine and the integration of inpatient and outpatient care through hospital-based medical practice will lead to more efficiency, higher quality care, and greater professional satisfaction.

Each of these ideas is worthy of extended discussion, but I am reluctant to delay the reader's direct encounter with Rorem. I will, therefore, limit my comment to only one of his themes—the potential conflict between physicians and hospitals for the health-care dollar. Writing in 1931, when third-party payment was rare, Rorem called attention to the "sharp competition for a share of the patient's resources." He went on to note that "the patient's ability to pay a certain doctor's fee may be directly influenced by his length of stay or type of accommodations in the hospital." With the growth of third-party reimbursement for the physician and the hospital, this competition, at least from the perspective of the physician, tended to disappear.

In the eighties, as the resistance to continued rapid expansion of health care expenditures grows, Rorem's original proposition will return in a new form. Presently it is not so much the individual patient who resists the growth of health care expenditures as it is the third party in either the public or private sector. In the next several years the government's contribution to health expenditures (almost half the total) will be restrained by opposition to higher taxes and by increasing competition for government funds (e.g., for defense, energy, the environment, and control of crime). There will also be increasing resistance in the private sector to ever higher health insurance premiums. In many local areas, employer groups are already forming to deal with health care costs.

One simple bit of arithmetic explains why resistance to the expansion of health care expenditures is likely to grow on both the public and private fronts. When the health sector represented only five percent of the GNP, an excess growth of health expenditures over GNP of two percent per annum implied a gain for the health sector of one percentage point (i.e., to six percent) in a decade. Now that the health sector is close to ten percent of the GNP, an identical gap of two percent per annum implies that the health sector captures an additional two percentage points of the GNP in the course of a decade. Because so much more is at stake now, the resistance on the part of those who must forego alternative uses of funds is likely to increase.

This slowing in the growth of health care expenditures will occur at a time when the number of physicians will be growing at a very rapid rate. Thus the tensions over the division of the pie are likely to be exacerbated. Expenditures per physician, it must be remembered, constitute the gross revenues of the physician, the hospitals, the drug companies, and other providers of medical goods and services. The physician's own revenues account for only a minor part of the total, but the physician's decisions have a great influence on the size of that total. Physicians, in their own self-interest, are likely to move toward modes of practice that hold down that portion of the expenditure package that finances hospitalization, drugs, and the like, rather than allow their own income to be reduced.

Many such modes of practice are already in place—prepaid group practice, independent practice associations, primary-care networks—and still others will be created in the years ahead. The central feature of all such modes is that the physician's own income is explicitly or implicitly tied to the total cost of care. The greater the expenditures for hospitals, drugs, and the like, the less is available for physician reimbursement. Physicians practicing in such modes are moved to re-examine their approaches to diagnosis and treatment in order to provide maximum care for their patients per dollar expended.

To be sure, there are potential problems with such modes, including the possibility of providing too little care. Moreover, the great majority of practicing physicians are comfortable with existing fee-for-service systems and will not eagerly accept such organizational changes. The logic and the force of external circumstances, however, are likely to prevail. This is exactly how Rorem saw the problem. In his 1950 paper advocating group practice, he wrote, "The sustaining motivation for physicians must be their personal self-interest, not social reform or demonstrations in medical economics. . . ."

For the most part, Rorem's critiques of health care and his vision of a better system seem to me to be right on the mark. If I have any reservation at all, it concerns a tendency in these articles to treat the utilization of care as purely a technological phenomenon. To the extent that Rorem believes that the amount of care is determined by "medical requirements," he does not do full justice to the effect of insurance on demand, or to the question of comparing marginal benefits and marginal cost. Fortunately, Rorem is still active and perhaps will address such questions in subsequent work. Meanwhile, his wisdom and humanity come through on every page of these selected papers. Rorem's work continues to be a source of inspiration and instruction to everyone involved in health care.

VICTOR R. FUCHS

The first essay in this selection was originally the final chapter of a 262-page volume entitled The Public's Investment in Hospitals, *published in 1930 by the University of Chicago Press. It was based upon visits, correspondence, and statistical analyses conducted over a period of two years, when I was an associate professor at the University of Chicago School of Business, and, later, a member of the research staff of the Committee on the Costs of Medical Care, Washington, D. C. The findings indicated that American hospitals were essentially social capital, provided by taxation and philanthropy without expectation of repayment or interest income. The report was summarized as Study No. 7 of the Committee. It suggested that interest and depreciation on capital investment be included in reimbursement formulas for health care financing. These suggestions later found expression in national public policy.*

Capital Investment and the Public

1. *Hospitals are, in the main, owned by the public.*—Ninety-one percent of the hospital capital has been provided by the public, without expectation of repayment or business return on the investment. The small amount invested in proprietary hospitals has been restricted to services for self-supporting individuals or groups. The physicians owning many of the small private hospitals declare that to a great degree these hospitals represent investments in private practice rather than hospitalization. If the hospital capital of the United States were to have been supplied by the approximately 140,000 physicians, there would have been required an initial investment of $22,000 each, and a current contribution from each of about $1,500 annually to make good depreciation. Less than 10 percent would ever have been repaid or have yielded an interest earning. These are the facts; the public owns the hospitals. The public, and not the medical professions or the patients through the payment of medical fees, has provided hospital capital. Is this an equitable distribution of this portion of the burden of hospitalization? Let us see.

What are the services of hospital capital, and who are the beneficiaries of this service? The patients who find their way to a hospital are, of course, the primary beneficiaries; but it is impossible to segregate from the general public those who will be patients and to ask them in advance for contributions to provide hospital plant and equipment. To be sure, proprietary hospitals achieve this result by giving services only to those who pay rates sufficient to recover all cost, including fixed charges. The money is advanced by business investors to provide the facilities for this small group.

But what should be done about the hospitalization of the general public? Many people requiring hospitalization are not able to pay for it in full, regardless of the reasons for their respective inabilities. Is it the responsibility of the medical profession to absorb part of the costs by erecting hospitals to be operated at a loss? Obviously not. Should the well-to-do patients of hospitals be assessed amounts sufficient to recover the losses incurred by serving patients whose payments do not cover the fixed charges? Many such patients have expressed their objection to such a policy by patronizing only hospitals where each patient pays his full share of the total costs. For well-to-do hospital patients to pay for free service to other members of the public is just as fair or unfair as for well-to-do patients of private physicians to be assessed higher fees for equivalent service because of a physician's charity work.

The services of capital investment must be regarded as accruing to all potential patients, not merely those who use its facilities. Even a wealthy patient cannot construct a hospital for his special needs after he has become ill. The hospital may be needed quickly, or not at all. It is in the interests of the public to have hospital facilities available for certain kinds of service, and the public must provide them. The public's interest in hospitalization is sufficient to justify governmental taxation and voluntary contributions as methods of providing capital investment. The fixed charges in this way are borne by the general public, and the operating costs alone may be assessed against patients as a class. But public policy has usually gone farther and approved a general levy on the community (either through governmental taxation or solicitation of voluntary contributions) for those patients who do not pay the full operating costs of their hospitalization, either because of unusually low economic status or because of the unusually expensive medical services needed. The responsibility for the payment of hospital costs incurred by patients unable to pay for themselves rests primarily with the general public and not with the medical professions or a small group of well-to-do patients. This responsibility, if recognized and met consistently, would avoid the necessity of "taxing" certain classes of patients through the medium of hospital fees. The policy of having one group of sick people contribute toward hospital care for others adds insult to injury, when one pauses to reflect upon the extent to which the incidence of diseases and conditions requiring hospitalization is the result of human relationships. One might as well say that the hospital bills should be paid only by the well members of the public.

2. *The public should exercise better control over its capital investment in hospitals.*—The general public which pays for its medical service, either through patients' fees or through compulsory or voluntary contributions, should be permitted to say whether, when, and where it will receive hospital care. The quality of the care is, of course, in the hands of physicians and the professions interested in hospitalization. But inasmuch as the public is providing the money for hospitals, it is entitled to control such expenditures. In a general way such control has been exercised through the activities of governmental units and through the co-ordination of nonprofit association policies, by the promotion of hospital councils, community chests, etc. But there is much left to be done in the co-ordination of the services of nonprofit association hospitals, which are peculiarly important because of the large number of patients using such hospitals for acute diseases and conditions.

Hospital care cannot, of course, be considered apart from its special role in complete medical care. It must be related to the number and training of the medical and nursing personnel, to the stage of development in public health, to the economic status and hygienic habits of the potential patients. Any community should view with alarm the expansion of hospital facilities, except in response to a recognized immediate or future need. It should not permit indiscriminate investment in hospital plant and equipment to satisfy racial, religious, social, or professional ambitions. Such action deprives the public of other benefits which might be of greater immediate or long-run value.

Capital investment should not exceed the limits of adequate medical service. Where it is permitted to transcend these limits, because of the demand for deluxe accommodations, the individual patients should pay the entire costs of the excess fixed charges thus incurred. The co-ordination of the total hospital facilities of a community is as important as flexibility of accommodations within the individual hospital. The hospital beds of a community are, of course, not always interchangeable. A bed in an asylum for nervous and mental cases is not available for a sick child. Likewise, a bed in a tuberculosis sanitarium is not available for a maternity case. Nevertheless, there are important advantages to be gained where hospitals co-ordinate their services, either by specializing on certain types of medical cases or by directing patients to hospitals where their special needs can be met most effectively.

3. *Control of capital investment financing policies has certain advantages and limitations.*—If a community were to budget its capital needs carefully, would not such a policy discourage large individual contributions? Possibly it would, especially if it were to rely heavily upon compulsory taxation. Moreover, it might remove some of the personal and human-

itarian element from the individual contributions, both large and small ones. On the other hand, controlled investment would assure meeting capital needs at the times they arose, and would avoid such an embarrassing situation as having to accept or reject offers which were inimical to the public welfare. It is possible, too, that many contributors would be glad to continue their large contributions, to be used in such manner as seemed most appropriate. These are practical matters which each community would need to consider when contemplating any program of controlling its hospital capital-investment program.

At present the capital requirements are irregular; but as hospital facilities improve, the capital needs will be limited to making good the depreciation of plant and equipment, with additional expenditures to keep pace with the growth of medical science and total increase in population if any. This new condition would lend itself to regular planning, and capital needs may be brought within the programs of community agencies supporting social services.

If community chests, and doctors and hospitals participating in their planning, were to change their policies and definitely set out to control hospital construction, and also to raise funds for plant and equipment, much good might be accomplished. The prevention of duplication of hospital facilities might release much capital for the current subsidizing of hospital care. This method is not in contemplation by most community chests and may not become an integral part of their policies within the near future.

4. *Costs of hospital services must be considered with relation to other medical services.*—Many illnesses do not require hospitalization, or require it only after long periods of self-treatment or physician's care in the home, accompanied by unemployment and expenses for additional help. These costs are all part of the costs of sickness, and the hospital patient may find that they amount to greater totals than the hospital bills. It does not suffice merely to reduce hospital costs while other expenditures continue or increase. Increased utilization of plant and equipment may result in lower fees for board-and-room service, even for diagnosis and therapy. But it does not provide sufficient funds for physicians' fees, special nursing services, the employment of maids in the home, or for the actual necessities of other members of the family. Hospital fees are only part of the total sickness bill, yet they usually are accompanied by other costs, and frequently follow a train of circumstances which make their payment difficult. Hospital service, being unusual, infrequent, and expensive, is not ordinarily included in the budgets of families which are otherwise self-supporting. Hospital costs often fall, therefore, with crushing weight upon already depleted fi-

nancial resources. It is because of this condition that much outcry is directed against hospital costs, although the amounts paid by individuals and the public to hospitals may be less than that for professional services or for drugs. Patients are interested in their total sickness bills, and a reduction of hospital fees to individual patients is only part of the cost of sickness, albeit an important one.

5. *Improved utilization of capital investment in government hospitals may release funds for the remuneration of professional groups.*—The payment of physicians for all work done for individual patients or for the public is an important feature of good hospitalization. There is no more reason for the medical profession to render free service in government hospitals than to assume the burden of expenditures for nurses, orderlies, or supplies. It has often been stated that physicians' personal services do not represent cash outlays for supplies, and hence are not of the same importance economically as other medical expenditures. But such is not the case. The only real distinction is historical, in that physicians in the past have been able to recover the value of their "donated" services by assessment against their full-pay patients, whereas nurses, orderlies, and the vendors of supplies have not been able to do so.

There is nothing inconsistent in a physician's receiving pay for service in a government hospital, where all other employees earn their livings by the work they do there, and when all groups participating in its construction have been remunerated on a business basis. In the past, to be sure, much medical care would probably have been impossible if physicians had not contributed their services to the care of patients in government hospitals. But it is undignified for an organized community to ask any group continually to make gifts of services or commodities to the public good without crediting them explicitly with their contributions. This custom must be regarded as a practical makeshift rather than a logical solution of the problem.

The situation with regard to nursing sisterhoods might be regarded as similar to that of physicians, except that members of the religious nursing orders have definitely withdrawn from the usual family life and are in all events assured of a livelihood, even though no personal wealth is accumulated. The public has never fully appreciated the extent of voluntary service which physicians, nuns, and deaconesses have rendered to the patients in American hospitals. The appropriate way in which the public should recognize the work of nursing sisterhoods is probably by more complete support in financing their hospitals. Physicians, however, are individually entitled to reasonable compensation for their services to government hospitals or to "free" patients under any and all conditions. The general public should pay the bill, and the physicians should not be required to charge such services to experience or advertising. Economies in hospital construction and the attendant reduction of fixed charges for hospital service will contribute toward this desirable objective.

The border line between nonprofit association hospitals and government hospitals is being gradually broken down. Governmental units are, on the one hand, contributing to the budgets of independent hospitals for the care of free patients; on the other hand, some government hospitals accept part-pay patients as well as full-pay patients who make payments to their private attending physicians. It is no disgrace at present to attend a public school or a state university. The time may come when an operation in a county hospital will be considered as respectable as one in a private hospital.

6. *The capital investment problem is not peculiar to hospitalization.*—All branches of medical and social service face the need for an understanding of the amount and significance of their capital investment. Most education costs are, of course, borne by the general public in the hope of an improved civilization. The "social capital" invested in the education of physicians, dentists, lawyers, clergymen, and teachers is very great. Heavy fixed charges result from the plant and equipment in medical schools, not to mention the investment made by the universities through the payment of the teaching staffs. These amounts, when added to the medical students' own expenditures during their course of study and internship, and their outlay for office equipment, make an imposing capital investment. A misunderstanding of the distribution of the fixed charges resulting from this capital investment lies at the root of much discussion and dissension concerning economic problems in private practice. A study of the capital investment by the general public and by the physicians in private or group practice might throw much light on the economic aspects of medical care.

7. *What of the future?*—The need for adequate utilization of capital investment is a pressing one at the present time. Will it become less acute in the near future? Probably not. The investment per bed in hospitals bids fair to increase for some time, possibly a decade, although there is some evidence that the total number of beds in the country may increase much more slowly. During 1929 nearly 1,000 hospital construction projects were undertaken, although during that year the total number of hospitals in existence remained practically stationary. The "registered" capacity increased by less than 15,000 beds, the growth resulting almost exclusively from the expansion of state nervous and mental hospitals. In the future hospital facilities will

doubtless continue to be improved, even if not enlarged in terms of bed capacity. Any solution of the problem must be found in the control of the capital investment rather than reducing it or retarding its growth. Even if the facilities were now satisfactory, there would still be needed annual expenditures of more than $100,000,000 to make good the depreciation. This means a contribution of nearly $1.00 per year for every man, woman, and child in America. At present the capital investment per person is approximately $25 per capita, not including endowment.

The capital investment problem is not the only one confronting hospitals at the present time. Much has been said by critics and defenders of present hospital service for and against the efficiency of management, the attitude of employees, the high intentions of boards of directors, the economy of labor and supplies, etc. The patient has been scored for his improvidence with regard to the burden of illness, his vanity in the selection of accommodations, his insistence upon unnecessary attention, and his irresponsible attitude toward the payment of hospital and physician's fees. All of these matters, important and interesting as they may be in the problems of medical costs, have been brushed aside in the foregoing discussion, in order that attention may be focused upon one single aspect of hospital service—capital investment and the fixed charges arising therefrom.

At the time the writer began this study, he felt that possibly one of the reasons for considering fixed charges was to establish a policy by which hospitals as a group could be self-supporting. The facts show that hospitals have never even approximated this condition. If the capital investment burden had not been carried by the general public, much hospital care could never have been rendered.

The nature of hospital service makes it essentially a public utility; and the burden of providing the capital investment should fall upon the ultimate beneficiary, the general public. But the problem of capital investment is not less important to individual hospitals by virtue of this fact. Careful analysis of fixed charges is required to place the burden upon the appropriate groups and to remove it from those who should not pay. A hospital should not assume that because fixed charges are not assessed against its patients, they are any the less actual "costs" to the general public which has provided the capital. Fixed charges are always present, and both hospital administration and financing require an appreciation of the role of capital investment in hospital care.

A private group clinic is an organization of health practitioners whose members cooperate professionally in service to individual patients. Several hundred were in existence in the West and Southwest in 1931, ranging in size from three to 300 participating doctors. My report of 125 pages was published in 1931 as Study No. 8 of the Committee on the Costs of Medical Care. The following statement was the preface to the second edition. Participants in private group clinics have increased more than tenfold during the past 50 years.

Private Group Clinics

The monograph *Private Group Clinics*, published in 1931, was a report describing a special method of providing medical care by groups of private practitioners. The study was conducted as part of a five-year program of the national Committee on the Costs of Medical Care. The analysis was based on typical examples of group practice in various parts of the United States, which by 1930 had attracted wide, but not always favorable, attention among the medical profession.

Group medical practice was considered by the Committee to be a significant special "experiment" in the provision of personal health service. The associated physicians used various names to identify themselves. They were called clinics, groups, services, foundations, or staffs, usually with a modifying term such as medical or surgical, a geographic area, or the names of one or more physicians.

The monograph was not intended to serve as a manual for medical administration, although the various chapters dealt with organization and management policies, property ownership, and public relations. Nor was the study a statistical appraisal of group medical practice. Although the analysis was essentially descriptive, it was incorporated with data derived from other studies of the Committee staff to formulate the first major recommendation contained in the Final Report, *Medical Care for the American People*, i.e., the encouragement of group practice nationally.

During the period of the study (1929 and 1930) there was no generally accepted definition of group medical practice, but the following features were considered characteristic: (1) physicians conduct their practice in a common facility; (2) physicians carry group responsibility for care of individual patients; (3) most physicians are full time with the group; (4) more than one medical specialty is represented within the group; (5) nonphysician business managers are engaged to handle administrative and financial aspects of the group; and (6) professional income is determined by mutual agreement rather than fees for services.

Throughout the years, the most important and controversial aspect of group medical practice has been the criterion that professional income would be distributed according to prior agreement among the member physicians.

At the time the *Private Group Clinics* study went to press the author's working definition had been formalized in the following words:

> A private group clinic is an organization of practitioners who engage jointly in medical practice from which results a single service to patients and a joint income to participating physicians and dentists. The clinic members offer service in more than one medical specialty, and usually provide all the diagnosis and therapy considered necessary for cases accepted by the group.

Thirty-five years later, the American Medical Association suggested the following definition for inclusion of organizations in *A Survey of Medical Groups in the United States, 1965:*

> Group medical practice is the application of medical services by three or more full-time physicians formally organized to provide medical care consultation, diagnosis and/or treatment through the joint use of equipment and personnel, and with the income from medical practice distributed in accordance with methods previously determined by the members of the group.

These definitions appear to emphasize organizational considerations for comparative purposes, but in its functional sense *group medical practice is a process, not a form of organization.* Group medical practice characterizes the full-time activities of many physicians employed by government agencies, business corporations, medical schools, hospitals, and other agencies. But the most widespread and significant form of group medical practice is the voluntary association of private practitioners who form partnerships or otherwise organize for the purpose of assuming joint responsibility for care of patients and for income distribution. Such physicians compete with solo practitioners and other clinics, but not with each other.

During the period of study available literature on group medical practice consisted of two short monographs, a fact that influenced both the scope and method of the study. Forty years later, the literature was increasing by more than 100 pages per month. A complete library on group medical practice would now comprise at least a 20-foot shelf of books, monographs, magazine articles, legislative reports, graduate study theses, and administrative manuals.

This preface makes no attempt to summarize developments in group practice during the past 40 years. It will be limited to some reflections and observations that appear relevant to the study of present-day group medical practice.

Group medical practice was described as an experiment 40 years ago by the Committee on the Costs of Medical Care, but the participating doctors would have rejected such a designation. Neither did they consider that they were conducting a "demonstration." They were merely trying to practice good medicine in a manner that gave them satisfaction and that recognized the social and professional forces affecting patient care.

Two general influences contributed to development of group medical practice in the 1930's. They are still important. The first was the development of "specialization" in business and professional activity, which created a need for coordination. The second factor was the increased reliance upon apparatus and equipment throughout society, including the delivery of health service. Modern equipment requires substantial capital investment, beyond the resources of most individual physicians or their capacity to use it effectively.

Group medical practice is an enlightened method of serving both professional and public interest. Some aspects of independence are surrendered when physicians agree to share responsibility and revenue. But the loss of independence is replaced by the special values of interdependence. The physicians are able to assist, advise, and substitute for each other when appropriate.

Group practice by physicians is the private counterpart of community planning for effective use of hospitals. The public investment in people deserves even more attention than its investment in buildings. In a broad sense, health practitioners are the "human" capital that is essential to *appropriate* use of buildings, equipment, and supplies. Group medical practice offers unique opportunities for recognizing and applying the standard of appropriateness to diagnosis, treatment, prevention, and rehabilitation.

As part of the study conducted 40 years ago, five questions were asked of physician members of 55 clinics and independent practitioners in the same communities. Written replies were obtained from several hundred practitioners. The questions referred to the following matters: the personal relationship between physician and patient; the effect of group medical practice activities upon local independent practice;

opportunities for research; suitability of clinic organization for general practice; and local professional encouragement or opposition.

Four decades ago physicians in group medical practice were not always accepted into the professional and social circles of their colleagues in their communities or throughout the nation. The opposition ranged widely in form, from intimations of unfair advantage, accusations of incompetence and interference with hospital staff appointments to denial of memberships in local professional societies. The situation appears to have changed materially. Members of medical groups increasingly are accepted into local medical societies and community hospital staffs.

Group medical practice is a method of providing personal health service that is independent of how patients served by the group finance the care they receive. Most private groups receive their income on the same basis and from the same sources as independent nongroup practitioners; that is, fees for services rendered as billed to individuals, Blue Shield or commercial insurance agencies, labor unions or industrial organizations, government agencies, and other private and public groups.

There has been a recent and continuing growth of consumer-sponsored group practice organizations by which medical groups agree to provide services to the members of specific organizations for stated annual fees per individual or family eligible to receive care. This arrangement has been referred to as *prepaid group practice*. The sponsoring organization may be the employees of a business enterprise, the members of a labor union, or individuals or groups in the general public who are enrolled through a special nonprofit corporation established for the purpose. Because group medical practice and prepayment have evolved separately a wide variety of interrelations has been demonstrated.

Certain numerical data and general facts about group practice situations in the years 1929 and 1930 appear in the monograph *Private Group Clinics*. Some are mentioned here as a matter of interest and for comparison with the present situation.

In 1930, about 150 multispecialty medical groups existed in the United States; they included about 1,800 physician members, with one organization reporting more than 200 doctors. Most of the clinics were in the middle west, in southern and western states and in towns of less than 50,000 inhabitants. Nearly all were organized as professional partnerships. A few clinics had formed corporations for the ownership of buildings or other legal transactions. A few clinics (about 15) owned hospitals. Others served as the closed staffs of certain hospitals. There were about two lay employees for each physician member. All clinics employed full-time business managers, none of whom participated in medical decisions or procedures.

The present scope of group practice is indicated by the findings of a *Survey of Medical Groups in the United States, 1965,* published by the American Medical Association in late 1968. There were estimated to be approximately 1,500 multispecialty groups, each with three or more members representing two or more medical specialties. These groups reported a total of about 17,000 member physicians in 1965, or about ten times the number estimated in the 1931 study.

The average number of physicians per group has increased during the years, with eight groups reporting 100 or more doctor members in 1965. Most of the larger groups own or control their own office space. About 90 groups engage in some degree of prepaid group practice.

The study also reported the existence of nearly 3,000 small groups composed exclusively of general practitioners or physicians practicing the same specialty, notably anesthesia, radiology, general surgery, obstetrics, or internal medicine. There was an average of four physicians per group; only a few such groups reported more than ten member doctors.

The 1931 monograph included a number of conclusions and predictions. Students of present day group medical practice may wish to compare the early appraisal with the situation in 1971. The 1931 conclusions and predictions were stated in essentially the following words:

Private group clinic physicians are in direct economic competition with other doctors in the same community. Their motive has been to practice medicine more effectively, not to reform the system for delivery of patient care.

The clinics exemplify the advantages of effective use of specialized personnel and facilities. Economies of scale are realized by full utilization of expensive equipment. There is opportunity for individual doctors to limit their work to their specialties.

Clinic physicians appear to recognize and respect the personal patient-physician relationship. Most clinics offer family-doctor services, and expect to maintain and expand these activities. Most clinics also expect to rely upon the recruitment of young doctors in expanding physician membership and professional services.

The average spendable income of physician members compares favorably with the earnings of independent practitioners in the same specialities. Operating costs are somewhat lower proportionately than in solo practice.

Private clinics are ideally structured to enter into annual contracts for prepaid group practice. Placement of business management in the hands of lay administrators frees the practitioners from such matters as accounting, pricing, insurance, purchasing, and personnel policies.

Group medical practice enables private clinic members to provide better care at lower costs than if they practiced as solo competitors. The profession faces the opportunity and the obligation to share these advantages with their patients and the general public.

Group medical practice does not require that all professional services be performed at one location. A number of clinics have established branch offices. Others maintain systematic relations with specialists in fields not represented in their membership.

Group medical practice is more than an administrative device to improve quality, to reduce costs to the public or to increase income of health practitioners. It is a way of life and an attitude toward health service. Its growth has been a process of evolution within medical practice following upon a revolution in medical science. As suggested 40 years ago, medical group practice is an enlightened and appropriate method of serving both professional and public interests.

The Taylor Society for the Advancement of Management held a symposium on hospital administration December 3, 1931 in New York City to which I contributed the following paper. It was based on findings presented to the Committee on the Costs of Medical Care and stressed the problems arising from interrelated and sometimes competitive professional activities at hospitals, namely, institutional care, private medical practice, and the activities of private-duty nurses. Some attention was also given to the patient's problem of paying for services, which are unpredictable and uncontrollable, and unrelated to ability to pay. The paper was published in the Bulletin *of the Taylor Society, February 1932.*

Some Economic Issues in Hospital Management

Hospitals are in many respects typical of all business enterprise. Procedures of scientific management in a hospital are much the same as those in a hotel or other place of business. But hospitals are also in some respects different from other business. The differences do not appear in the detailed procedures, but in those phases of scientific management concerned with the "policies" of the institution as a whole. It is important to recognize certain economic aspects of hospital service if the public is to understand the problems confronting the directors of hospitals, and if the hospital administrators themselves are to direct their institutions to the best advantage.

I

Hospital services must be sharply differentiated economically from certain other types of medical care rendered in the hospital buildings. Hospital care itself includes several distinct services for which the patients pay separate fees. The distinctive hospital product is the service usually referred to as "board and room," which includes the use of a bed, three meals per day, and, within certain limits, the ministrations of graduate or student nurses. It is the board-and-room service for which a patient pays his room rate of five dollars or eight dollars per day. Other important products of a hospital are X-ray services, laboratory services, and other diagnostic or therapeutic procedures. An increasing number of institutions are also providing office care to patients who are "up and about." Each hospital service is usually charged for as a separate hospital product, if charged for at all.

But there are also other economic and professional activities in the hospital which are not ordinarily under the hospital's direct control. The services of attending physicians and surgeons are not usually considered as hospital products. Doctors have been regarded as conducting their own businesses when dealing with their private patients in hospitals. They form their business relationships with such patients with little or no knowledge or supervision on the part of the hospital superintendent. Likewise, when additional nursing service beyond that included in board and room is required, the "special nurse" and the patient effect financial dealings independent of the hospital authorities. The hospital building, therefore, may serve to house three independent business entities—that of the hospital, the doctor and the special nurse. Each separate professional service is purchased and paid for independently by the patient. Only the "hospital" services, as such, come under the direct supervision and financial control of the superintendent.

At one time all financial problems of services in the hospitals were controlled by the institutions themselves. Only nonpaying patients were accepted, most of them being admitted for isolation rather than to improve professional care. But the hospitals have changed from hospices for the poor or hopelessly sick; they are now workshops for carrying on the highest type of professional activity. When private self-supporting patients were first admitted to hospitals, they were introduced as guests by the physicians of the community. The hospitals accepted these *paying* patients as a courtesy to the medical staff who attended the *free* patients. The policy of selling as well as donating hospital services was thus entered upon by inviting the medical and nursing professions to attend their paying patients within the institutions. The hospitals' financial dealings with private patients, originally few in number, were, of course, limited to the services rendered by the hospital personnel and facilities. At the present time the paying patients of private physicians have become the most important source of the revenue for the hospitals of the United States.

The independence of the hospital, the physician and the special nurse, each charging separate fees, at times results in sharp competition for a share of the patient's resources, for the patient's ability to pay a certain doctor's fee may be directly influenced by his length of stay or type of accommodations in the hospital. Likewise, the substantial fees required for special-nursing service may make exceedingly difficult the payment of either a hospital bill or doctor's bill. The hospital superintendent, therefore, is not able to regard his product as an independent commodity merely to be delivered to and paid for by his customer.

Hospital care to paying patients is usually delivered along with an economically competing product, namely, the services of an attending doctor or a special nurse.

Some hospitals are making an effort to co-ordinate to some degree all financial relations with patients. One institution has inaugurated a middle-rate plan by which physicians' fees are limited in amount for patients occupying certain types of room accommodations, and by which special-nursing service is permitted only on recommendation of the attending doctors and the hospital authorities. A number of other hospitals, particularly those connected with universities, have engaged full-time doctors who serve as representatives of the hospital and who attend all patients accepted by the institution. The hospitals thereby tend to become medical centers offering various types of professional services, rather than mere buildings in which independent professional activities are performed. Such policies of co-ordination, if developed more widely, would do much to clarify and aid in the solution of problems of hospital management and economic policy.

II

Most hospitals have been constructed and equipped by the general public, who have contributed funds for the purpose either voluntarily or through taxation. Hospital plant and equipment are usually financed on a nonprofit basis, without expectation of repayment of principal to, or the receipt of earnings by, the individual investors. Even in those cases where hospital bonds are issued by a private charitable institution or a government, it is usually expected that the interest payments or ultimate redemption of the debt will be accomplished by voluntary contributors or tax-payers rather than by the hospital's earnings from the sales of its product. The hospital superintendent, therefore, conducts his business with a publicly owned plant and equipment.

The fact that most hospital service is conducted with capital supplied by the community has influenced hospital management in several ways. It has tended to obscure in the minds of some hospital superintendents the existence of the overhead costs of interest and depreciation. In those cases where allowances for interest and depreciation need not be recorded to balance the cash expenditures of the hospital, some hospital directors appear to have forgotten that plant and equipment represent important economic outlays from which the public has a right to expect the greatest possible professional benefit. The ordinary hospital ledger of accounts contains no allowance for depreciation or interest on the investment in plant and equipment.

If this omission had its influence merely upon the ledger, the practice would be of no great importance. It would be a matter of interest only to accountants, who might then argue over the problem. But when a community donates $500,000 or a million dollars to build, equip or endow a hospital, it withdraws that money from other public or private enterprise. The money invested in a hospital, which will last thirty or fifty years, cannot be recalled and subsequently invested in a playground, a church, a milk fund or in a profitable business. Interest and depreciation are actual costs to the community of hospital service, even though these "fixed charges" may be paid in advance through public provision of plant and equipment.

An analysis of the total costs of hospital service reveals that the fixed charges per patient day may range from fifty cents to five dollars depending upon the degree to which beds are occupied and upon the relative amounts of investment per bed. It is important that hospital superintendents realize the tremendous waste of public funds when hospital rooms and scientific apparatus remain idle for want of an administrative policy which would bring them into public service. The recognition of fixed charges as costs of hospital care does not mean that patients' fees should necessarily be established at levels sufficient to recover allowances for interest and depreciation. This recognition may, in fact, merely serve as the basis for removing the burden of fixed charges from certain classes of patients. The important thing is to recognize the responsibility for adequate use of the publicly owned plant and equipment. The benefits of the public's investment in hospitals can be realized fully only when the plants are utilized to the greatest degree consistent with good professional care.

The superintendent of a hospital is not always responsible for the inadequate utilization of plant and equipment. He may be in charge of an institution built without regard to the needs of the community, planned without regard to economies in operation, or erected merely as a lavish monument to a wealthy donor. A public awareness of the place of fixed charges in hospital costs, and of the influence of plant and equipment upon other operating costs, would tend to discourage unnecessary, poorly planned, or elaborate hospitals. As a result, existing institutions would reap economies from quantity production, and hospital managers would have access to additional community funds for the payment of operating costs. Some hospital directors and trustees are fully aware of the importance of fixed charges in hospital financing and costs, but the subject still requires careful study and attention.

III

Medical care—including hospital care—is regarded by the public not only as an economic commodity, but also as a philanthropic service. For patients able to purchase and pay for hospital care, the product of a hospital is expected to be supplied at a price equal to its full cost of production, including fixed charges. Other members of the population are expected to receive hospital care free or at fractions of the total costs of the various services they require. The superintendent who delivers hospital care free to patients turns for repayment to the financially able members of the general public. These persons are expected to finance the free care of others through paying fees which yield net surpluses, or through voluntary or tax contributions. As a rule, a hospital finds the revenue from paying patients insufficient to cover the total operating costs of the institution's services (even when fixed charges are excluded from the calculation).

The social policy of attempting to provide hospital care according to a patient's need rather than his pocketbook is the cause of much confusion in the public mind with regard to hospital efficiency. Daily room-rates of hospitals are compared with those of hotels, with the implication that if hotels can be managed with profit to the owners, hospitals should at least be self-supporting. There are, of course, very few hotels which could meet their operating costs if from one-third to one-half of the guests paid nothing at all, or amounts substantially below the costs of the services they received. It takes money to pay expenses, and if patients cannot pay the costs of services they require, the superintendent should have authority to do one of two things—to refuse such patients admittance to his hospital or to demand adequate payment by the public for all services rendered to its individual members.

A deficit may result either from excessive expenditures or inadequate receipts. Expenditures are in large part under the superintendent's control and he should be expected to reduce them to the minimum. Receipts are also in large part under the superintendent's control, and he should be expected to keep them at the maximum consistent with the public policy adopted by the trustees and the hospital's supporters. But when the public demands that care be given to its individual members, it should also guarantee adequate payment, and should not place the responsibility of financing such service entirely upon the superintendent's shoulders.

The superintendents of hospitals are in part responsible for misunderstandings of hospital financing methods. They have allowed their need for public support to be referred to as "operating deficits" instead of as "costs of services" rendered to the general public. The difference between operating costs and patients' fees may be regarded merely as a statement of the costs of professional services rendered to the public—a bill which the community should expect to pay promptly and in full. To the extent that such a bill appears unduly large, it should be scrutinized with care. It is the superintendent's obligation to remove from the community any portion of the economic burden resulting from his own inefficiency. But it is the public's responsibility to remove from the superintendent that portion of the economic burden resulting from the community's demands for hospital care or from an unwise investment of that community in plant and equipment.

IV

A carefully planned system of cost analysis would be of immense benefit to a superintendent, not only in the control of hospital expenditures, but also in the enlistment of public support. Hospital service, as has been stated, is not a homogeneous product. Some departments are self-supporting from patients' fees. Some are not. If the total costs of each hospital service were determined separately, such calculations would show clearly the need or opportunity for economies from increased utilization of hospital facilities. Unit costs could be calculated for board-and-room care, X-ray services, laboratory tests, etc., and these costs then compared with existing fees. The comparison would permit the establishment of fees intended to yield the greatest surplus or the minimum loss from certain services. It may prove, for example, that a lowering of the fees for X-ray services would result in such an increased demand that unit costs would be materially reduced.

The public's interest in hospital care requires that some fees be established at levels presumed to cover only portions of their respective costs. The very low daily rates in most hospital "wards"—two dollars or three dollars—are evidence of this public policy, for these rates are presumed to be lower than the costs of the services to which they apply. The ward rates are established at these levels for the purpose of allowing certain members of the population to benefit from the public's voluntary and tax contributions, but also to pay sums within the limits of their reasonable ability to pay. The data from an analysis of hospital costs would enable the hospital superintendent to show clearly which of the various services were not self-supporting from patients' fees. For example, one hospital's entire need for public support may result from the inadequate fees collected for board-and-room care in the wards or from outpatient care. In another institution the need for public funds may be traceable directly to the costs of education for student nurses. But it should be made clear that community support of hospitals is, properly considered, merely the payment of a bill for important public services and not a subsidy for poorly trained hospital administrators.

V

In the popular sense of the term patients never "demand" hospital service, in the sense that they prefer it to automobiles, clothes, or radios. On the other hand, when a patient is in need of hospital care, he demands it without delay or regard to price. The service *must* be bought, else the patient *may* never buy again. Expenditures for hospital service are usually compulsory, even though the patient himself may not expect or be able to bear the burden.

In addition to being compulsory, expenditures for hospital service are irregular and unanticipated. No one knows exactly when he will require hospital care, yet everyone knows that he probably will require it at some time. A large group of individuals can do what it is impossible for one individual to accomplish. The group can predict approximately the total hospital care the members will require during a given period of time, also the total expenditures which will be necessary on their behalf. Some patients will require services priced at five or ten dollars, others at several hundreds of dollars. Some will receive no hospital service. The group can budget the amount and costs of hospital care to the entire number, but no individual can anticipate the time or amount of an expenditure on his own behalf.

Hospital service is generally a part of a "high cost" illness. Usually hospitalization comes at the end of previous treatment, which may have involved expenses for physicians and nurses, absence from gainful employment, and frequently expenditures for help in the home. A ten-day stay in the hospital almost never causes total expenditures of less than $50, and they frequently exceed $100. A study of 10,000 cases by Messrs. McNamara and Parker showed average hospital fees of $77 in one hundred hospitals in 1929. Such an average is not a staggering amount, and if a person could be assured that his hospital bill would never exceed this average and would come with regularity, he probably could budget for such hospital care. But the hospital bill itself for a serious condition requiring major surgery is probably not more than half of the total expenditures. Other outlays are required for medical attendance, and for special nursing. Absence from gainful employment usually swells the net economic loss from illness to much higher totals.

Moreover, no family can be sure, after it has paid a total hospital and medical bill of $300 or $500, that it will not be called upon to do so again in the near future.

Hospitalized cases, therefore, are not to be considered in the same economic class as cases of minor illnesses, during which a patient may continue in a gainful occupation and for which he may from time to time pay relatively small fees for professional services or for drugs and medicines. Every hospitalized illness is an exceptional case, from the standpoint of the individual, and the financing of hospital care, therefore, cannot be accomplished by the same methods as suffice for simple illnesses.

Summary

Hospital service is similar in many details to other types of business. The economic policies now current in hospital service, however, create special problems which make hospital administration unique, complex, and difficult.

First, hospital care is usually delivered in conjunction, and frequently in economic competition, with a doctor's or special nurse's services.

Second, hospital service is conducted with the use of community capital, donated without expectation of repayment or of interest earnings. This fact has tended to obscure the role of fixed charges in hospital costs, also the economic advantages of adequate utilization of plant and equipment. The public's method of investing in hospitals has at times burdened efficient superintendents with the management of institutions which were unnecessary for a community's needs or which were so poorly planned as to interfere with economical administration.

Third, hospital service is in part regarded by the public as a social service to be provided without regard to ability to pay. Fees have usually not been established with a view to recovering the full costs of the services, and many individual patients pay little or nothing for hospital care.

Fourth, analysis of the costs of hospital service would be desirable as a basis both for efficiency and for adequate financing, for, if fees are to be kept low by public policy, the cost analysis provides the explanation of the need for public support and sets forth a detailed statement of hospital services for the general public. Cost analysis from this point of view would be an aid to financing, as well as to internal efficiency of administration.

Fifth, hospitalized illnesses, because of their irregularity and their relatively high costs, can be budgeted by the individual only through some type of insurance. There can be no adequate support from patients' fees until it is possible for individuals to budget the cost of their hospital care from year to year. This requirement involves a system of group responsibility for hospital care by which individuals may insure the hospital and the medical profession for the payment of their medical bills. Just what form this insurance should take is not the immediate problem, but if the patient of moderate means is ever to be self-supporting with regard to hospital care, it must be possible for him to budget hospital service along with other necessities.

The next essay was presented at the Annual Congress on Medical Education and Hospitals of the American Medical Association, Chicago, February 15, 1932. I was invited to the Congress while serving as a staff member of the Committee on the Costs of Medical Care. The essay stresses the central role of physicians in health care at hospitals and applauds the instances where physicians carry on private office practice there. The public is well served when doctors see their vertical and horizontal patients at the same location; the doctor is always "in." Moreover, the physician is able to give more attention to those under his supervision.

The Hospital as a Medical Service Center

It has been my privilege during the last three years to be in almost continuous contact with physicians and hospital administrators. This experience has convinced me that if the people of the United States have not at all times and places received good medical care the fault does not lie in the lack of scientific knowledge or skill on the part of the medical profession, or in the lack of a willingness to serve on the part of the average individual practitioner. The difficulty is to be found rather in the failure to transmit the benefits of medical knowledge and skill according to a plan which is satisfactory to both physicians and patients.

The physician is logically the central figure in the prevention and care of illness. The benefits from the physician's scientific training and professional activities can be realized, however, only when other medical personnel and facilities are co-ordinated with the services of the doctor of medicine. Pharmacists, nurses, medical technicians, and lay assistants are secondary practitioners, and their activities should at all times serve to extend the physician's influence and to increase the benefits from his activities. No physician, and very few subordinate medical practitioners, would be likely to deny the validity of this principle. Yet the facts reveal that much medical service is not conducted in such a way as to pass on to the public the maximum benefits from the physician's knowledge and skill.

I wish to suggest to you one method by which the physicians may increase the value of their services to the public, and by which doctors and patients may derive both professional and financial benefits. The method is not a new one; it is already in operation by many practitioners in the United States. It consists in the greater use of hospitals, personnel, and facilities in the treatment of ambulatory private cases. This procedure does not mean that the hospital will tend to control the practice of medicine. In fact, it brings the practice of medicine even more completely under the doctor's own auspices. The doctor uses the hospital as the instrument for conserving his energies and extending his influence.

The typical modern hospital for the treatment of acute medical and surgical cases contains the scientific apparatus and equipment necessary for the diagnosis and treatment of cases which are admitted. In addition the hospital includes nurses, technicians, and other personnel well-trained and disciplined in the medical services recommended or prescribed by physicians. An entire hospital staff may, generally speaking, be regarded as physicians' assistants in the care of patients admitted to the institution. These assistants make possible the treatment of many patients who could not be served if physicians were to perform the various detailed activities themselves.

The benefits of a hospital—that is, of well-trained personnel and adequate scientific apparatus—are shared by all economic groups of the general public, and by all physicians who attend cases receiving bed care. These professional and economic advantages, regularly utilized in the care of inpatients, have prompted the development of outpatient services in a great many institutions. The hospital, with apparatus and personnel available, has co-operated with the physician in the care of free and part-pay patients by conserving the doctor's time and by supplementing his personal services to these patients. Many physicians, accordingly, have tended to concentrate their services to nonpaying ambulatory cases in the outpatient departments of the hospitals where they attend their private patients requiring bed care. Hospitals with outpatient departments are to a degree medical-service centers for the physicians who utilize them and for the patients eligible to receive treatment at the institutions.

But there are, generally speaking, many doctors and patients who do not receive the benefit of the available hospital personnel and apparatus. Some physicians have no regular hospital affiliations, and even the doctors who hold hospital appointments do not ordinarily use the institution in the treatment of office cases. The entire facilities of a hospital are utilized when necessary in the treatment of bed patients, regardless of their financial status. But physicians often refrain from the use of hospital personnel and apparatus in the treatment of ambulatory patients if these patients are considered able to pay private fees for their medical care. In private office practice, therefore, doctors ordinarily rely upon such personnel or apparatus as they maintain in their own offices, or refer their private patients to other practitioners, commercial laboratories, or technicians who specialize in the services necessary to diagnosis or therapy.

Doctors, hospitals, and patients would benefit greatly if physicians and surgeons used more generally the personnel and equipment of hospitals in the treatment of their private-office cases, and did not restrict such procedure to the care of bed cases and of the poor admitted to the outpatient departments. The development of this practice would not involve a revolutionary procedure, for a substantial minority of the medical profession have already availed themselves of the opportunities which hospitals offer in this respect. The custom has been quietly growing in recent years in many communities, and at present several thousand doctors rely upon hospital personnel and apparatus in a part or all of their private-office practice. Before discussing the advantages and limitations of this procedure, I will outline some of the ways in which physicians have been using hospitals in diagnosis and therapy for private ambulatory patients.

There are in the United States about two thousand registered hospitals owned by physicians, either individually or in groups. These hospitals are mostly small ones—in fact, they comprise less than 10 percent of the hospital-bed capacity of the United States. But the majority of these institutions contain more complete scientific apparatus and equipment than the individual physicians could have maintained in their private offices. Some physicians maintain their private offices in the hospital building, these doctors being the ones financially and professionally responsible for the activities of the institution as a whole. The physicians owning hospitals usually consider the institutions as adjuncts of their private practice rather than as separate organizations. Both full-pay and charity cases present themselves at the doctors' offices, and, as a rule, there is no separate outpatient department for free or part-pay cases. Doctors owning shares in the hospital, but not maintaining offices in the institution, rely upon the X-ray and laboratory facilities for the care of private-office cases.

A number of teaching hospitals connected with university medical schools have in recent years provided offices that faculty members may use in the treatment of their private cases. Usually these offices are separate from the outpatient department in which free or part-pay cases are attended as part of the instruction of medical students or interns. Outstanding examples of this arrangement are the Medical Center affiliated with Columbia University and the hospitals of Western Reserve University. A somewhat different arrangement prevails in those teaching hospitals served by salaried physicians and surgeons who comprise the entire faculty of the medical schools and the entire attending staffs for outpatient and inpatient service. These doctors accept private patients on behalf of the university medical schools and hospitals. Well-known institutions using this arrangement are the Universities of Chicago, Iowa, and Michigan.

There appears to be a tendency for community hospitals which maintain outpatient departments for free or part-pay cases to allow certain attending physicians occasionally to see private patients either before or after the regular hours during which the various clinics are open to the public. Data accumulated by the statistical department of the Council on Medical Education and Hospitals indicate that several hundred institutions in the United States permit some physicians to attend private ambulatory patients in the hospitals. The nature of these privileges, as to the number of physicians or the types of cases, varies with the hospital extending them. The preliminary data, however, indicate a growing tendency for individual institutions to encourage some private-office practice in the hospital.

A number of nonprofit association hospitals have sponsored the construction of physicians' office buildings adjacent to the main hospital structure, and connected by halls or underground passageways. Office space is rented to the individual doctors, and the scientific apparatus and equipment of the hospital are utilized in the treatment of private-office cases at agreed fees. Physicians rely almost entirely upon the equipment of the hospital for the diagnosis and treatment of difficult cases, in this way reducing the overhead costs of maintaining their respective private offices.

In a large southern city approximately one hundred physicians occupy offices in a building constructed adjacent to one of the large hospitals. A medium-sized hospital in Chicago has erected a building in which ten private specialists are located. In a Wisconsin city a hospital conducted under religious auspices provided temporary quarters for a group of fourteen doctors whose building had been destroyed by fire. The temporary arrangement proved so satisfactory to doctors, hospital, and patients that it has been continued for more than five years.

The Duke Endowment, in drawing its model plans for small hospitals, has made it possible for local physicians to maintain their private offices in the main hospital building. When only four or five doctors are situated in a town, this arrangement also makes unnecessary the construction of a separate outpatient department for nonpaying cases, since the office practice at the hospital may include the care of such patients. In a small New Hampshire town the three doctors of the community have recently established their offices in a wing of the local hospital, paying an agreed rental to the institution for the use of the examining and consulting rooms.

A community hospital in a Massachusetts town of three thousand serves a rural area in which twenty-two doctors are located. Physicians in outlying villages are encouraged to bring their private-office cases to the hospital for study, and are allowed to use the examining rooms of the outpatient department without charge to themselves or their patients. None of the physicians in the area maintains offices in the institution. During the investigator's visit, a doctor from a village nine miles distant was at the hospital, and received a call from his office saying that a patient awaited him there. The patient decided, at the suggestion of the physicians, to come to the hospital for examination, thereby saving the need for a special trip later, in case X-ray or laboratory service were necessary.

The medical profession is familiar with the organization of the several hundred private-group clinics in the United States, some of which own or conduct hospitals as private ventures or use almost exclusively the medical apparatus and facilities of one or two existing hospitals. In every instance the group of physicians have arranged in their purchase of scientific apparatus and equipment to avoid duplication of the facilities in their offices with that available in the hospitals which they use for inpatient care. In a few cases the private-group clinics rent space from independent hospital associations and conduct their office practice in a special wing or floor of the hospital set aside for this purpose. Two well-established nonprofit association hospitals in the East, one in Pennsylvania and one in Massachusetts, have erected clinic buildings for groups of about twenty physicians, who pay regular rental for the office space and utilize the hospital facilities in the treatment of all cases.

A less intensive type of service, though one which is becoming more common in the United States, is the arrangement by which independent practitioners utilize the pathological and X-ray laboratories of the hospital to supplement their office facilities. An increasing number of hospitals offer service to individual practitioners in the treatment of their cases, charging the appropriate fees either to the attending physician or directly to the patients treated. A well-known hospital in Chicago which maintains no outpatient department nevertheless renders a large volume of X-ray service for the private-office cases attended by staff physicians. Several of the staff attend private-office cases in the hospital, but a large number of them use the X-ray department, as well as the laboratories, in the diagnosis and treatment of private-office cases.

Enough illustrations have been cited to indicate a definite trend toward private-office practice in the hospitals of the United States. What are the advantages and limitations of this procedure from the point of view of the medical profession, the hospitals, and the patients? The private physician, whether or not he maintains an office within the hospital, has the advantage of continuously available professional personnel and scientific apparatus. If he uses an office within the hospital, on either a full-time or a part-time basis, he gains from frequent contacts with other physicians whose judgment or services may be needed in diagnosis or therapy. The expense for office space in a hospital would be lower than for equivalent facilities obtained individually. Physicians could utilize common waiting rooms and office and technical personnel, thereby reducing important overhead costs in the conduct of their practice. When desirable, a group of independent physicians could engage a layman to supervise certain administrative and financial details of their activities. The physicians could, if they wished, co-operate in the maintenance of case records, not to mention their opportunities to substitute for and assist one another during emergencies, vacation periods, or absences at professional meetings.

The hospitals also would gain by a closer affiliation with private physicians in the treatment of office cases. Personnel and equipment would be used to a greater capacity. Technical services would be maintained at a high professional level through contact with and scrutiny by the physicians. Patients would become used to attendance at a hospital and more inclined to use its facilities when in need of bed care. In addition to co-operating with private physicians, the hospital might also become the center of the public-health activities of its locality. The benefits of the public's investment in hospitals, whether erected from voluntary contributions or tax funds, would thus be made available to a larger proportion of the community. For the private-office cases of physicians are greater in number than the hospitalized illnesses and the patients treated in outpatient departments combined.

Individual patients might save much time through private-office practice in the hospital, particularly if there were need of consultation with several physicians. Moreover, a patient's personal physician could more easily co-ordinate the findings of the various specialists and technicians than if they were located in entirely separate offices.

The objections to an increase of office practice in the hospital, and the co-ordination of medical services which would result therefrom, are the same objections that may be raised against co-ordinated practice generally. There is the possibility that physicians might be deprived of certain professional prerogatives, that the personal relationship between doctor and patients might be diminished, and that the readily available scientific apparatus might encourage unnecessarily elaborate diagnosis and therapy. These dangers are, of course, also possible in independent private practice, without the offsetting advantage to the patient of conserving his time in the search for medical care or to individual physicians of being able to check any commercial tendencies which might dominate the practice of other independent physicians or surgeons. It may be objected that there is not room for all American physicians in the existing hospital plant and equipment. The objection is a valid one, and, if all doctors were immediately to apply for office space in the hospitals of the United States, they would not merely tax the capacity of existing hospitals, but also require the construction of additional buildings. In some communities, moreover, the location of certain of the existing hospitals would not be convenient for the office practice of their staffs.

There is little probability that private-office practice will shift to hospitals with such rapidity as to embarrass hospital superintendents and trustees. Nevertheless, the centering of medical service in the hospital, which already represents an important concentration of capital investment and professional personnel, would appear to have great practical advantages for doctors, hospitals, and patients. Physicians and hospitals, particularly in small communities, may well co-operate in the conduct of their private-office practice, and hospital trustees will do well to provide office facilities for attending physicians. The hospital as a medical-service center is the logical development of the need for coordinating the medical personnel and facilities of a community and for increasing the influence and leadership of the medical profession in the care and prevention of illness.

The following paper was presented at the annual conference of State Medical Association Secretaries and Editors, Chicago, November 1949, and published in Trustee, *February 1950. At the time I was director of the Hospital Council of Philadelphia. Hospitals and doctors are not in competition. The courts have decreed that hospitals cannot practice medicine for the simple reason that a corporation cannot enroll in a medical school. Physicians may legally own hospitals. Hospitals may legally employ physicians. But health care will always be a unified process from the patient's point of view.*

Inseparable Team: Physician and Hospital

A clear professional distinction between present-day medical practice and hospital service has become impossible. The old-time hospital was essentially a custodial institution for people considered a menace to the public health or a disturbance to the peace and safety of the community. Medical practitioners' contracts with these hospitals were intermittent, and were incidental to the main function of board and room service.

But the situation has changed greatly. Medical service now is regarded as the central purpose of all the activities conducted within a hospital. Services of diet and custody are incidental to the planned functions of diagnosis and treatment. In fact, many patients do not remain long enough to enjoy the hospitality of bed and board services, which originally were the essential features of the institution.

Medical service is a professional, not an economic, concept. The professional distinction between medical practice and hospital service disappears completely when physicians accept full-time salaries for their work in hospitals, or when groups of doctors cooperate with each other in the formation of clinics for full-time or part-time practice of medicine in hospitals.

Legal distinctions between medical practice and hospital service are likewise difficult to establish. Hospital trustees and management can arrange to provide the medical services of licensed physicians for patients, and many have done so, particularly in the various diagnostic specialities. Obviously the hospital cannot practice medicine. It is impossible to detect a heart murmur with a bedpan or swab a throat with a slide rule.

The courts have reiterated the stand that hospitals cannot practice medicine, not because it is in violation of law, but because it is contrary to observable fact. Legal controversies over corporate practice of medicine have invariably centered upon the contractual arrangements for providing medical service rather than legal permissibility for an institution to diagnose and treat patients. Medical practice must be performed by a physician or under his supervision. A hospital is one of the places where medical practice occurs.

A patient pays his bill from a single bank account and he experiences his suffering within the confines of a single mind and body. The conventional practice of separating the costs of a hospitalized illness into payments of physicians' services, hospital services, and private nursing services is confusing and unsatisfactory. Wherever patients are given an opportunity to budget their total sickness costs as a single item, they invariably welcome the privilege, with resulting increased security to the medical practitioners and institutions.

One example of this fact is the popularity of hospitals in which medical fees are established in advance on the basis of the character of the professional procedure rather than the individual's presumed or actual ability to pay. Another example is the rapid growth of prepayment plans in which medical fees and hospital bills are a single benefit, rather than separate and competing forms of insurance protection.

Many doctors depend primarily for their livelihood upon work performed in hospitals. This applies particularly to specialists in the field of surgery, and also to physicians in the various diagnostic specialties which require the use of apparatus and equipment. Conversely, the income of most voluntary hospitals is directly influenced by the physicians who bring patients to these institutions. The medical staff determine which patients will be hospitalized, and they determine what services will be performed in their behalf. Thus, medical practitioners also affect the expenses of the institution.

One factor in the present high costs of care in hospitals is the demand by physicians that certain types and quantities of diagnostic procedures be performed in behalf of their patients. Unnecessary services provided on a doctor's recommendations may reduce a patient's ability to pay a reasonable professional fee for the personal services of that physician.

It is the responsibility of hospital business management to carry out necessary procedures with a minimum of expenditure for supplies and personal services. It is the responsibility of medical practitioners to request professional and institutional services for their patients in accord with medical requirements, knowing that the full costs ultimately must be paid by the patients and the general public.

Physicians and hospitals thus are natural allies in the war on disease. Some persons would make it appear that they are natural enemies in a struggle for control over medical practice. Physicians already control the scientific and professional phases of medical practice. This can never be taken from them, even if lay groups ever would attempt such action.

But the economic aspects of medical practice in hospitals are the joint responsibility of physicians, trustees, and management. The doctors control the professional work. The trustees and management are responsible for seeing that patients finance the cost of the services they receive, either as individual patients who receive care or as potential patients in the role of Blue Cross subscribers, insurance policyholders, taxpayers, or philanthropists.

Specialized practice in hospitals differs from general practice in homes in one very important respect. Usually the general practitioner is acquainted with the patients who seek his advice; if not, he finds occasion to learn something of each patient's environment and to adjust the treatment and charges to the family pocketbook. But at the present time, general medical practice represents only fifteen cents of each dollar spent for various types of health services.

Many specialists are not personally acquainted with the patients for whom they perform very important services. Neither the general practitioner nor the specialist can control the prices which must be charged to meet the costs of dentistry, drugs, custodial service, or nursing care. Only one sickness out of ten requires hospitalization, but such illnesses are the source of 50 per cent of the income of the total medical profession.

American hospitals and the American medical profession therefore will share the same destiny. Intelligent cooperation among physicians, hospital trustees, and hospital management can shape the form of medical service for generations to come. If these groups waste their energies by conflict they will invite public control of a type which may stifle scientific spirit and managerial efficiency.

Some physicians have said that they fear the trustees of a voluntary hospital more than the bureaucracy of a governmental agency. In my opinion, this point of view is short-sighted and gives undue emphasis to momentary but solvable problems.

Hospital trustees are prompted solely by a desire to serve their communities and, in most instances, are influenced by proposals from the medical profession. If trustees have, from time to time, unduly interfered with the quality and character of medical practice in their institutions, the cause may be traceable to the absence of alternative suggestions by the staff which were capable of fulfillment. In the final analysis, hospital trustees are responsible for the total hospital services provided.

Regardless of the emotional tensions which may have developed in some institutions and communities, the hospital is still the doctor's best friend. It is an essential instrument for the application of specialized knowledge and skill, without which many of the gains of modern medical science could not be realized, and without which the practice of many individual professional men would not go forward satisfactorily.

In the "cold war" which exists in some areas between hospitals and doctors, both sides will lose. The doctors will lose their present degree of independent action and the public will lose its sense of participation in the program of health conservation and personal welfare. No layman, whether he be hospital administrator, trustee, or patient, need apologize for expressing an intense interest in the organization and financing of hospitals. Both groups have the same objective, namely, the best possible health service, at the lowest possible cost, with the greatest sense of personal participation by doctor and patient. It is the privilege of hospital representatives to recognize this goal and to cooperate with doctors in working toward its fulfillment.

Group Medical Practice is a process in health care, not a form of organization. It may occur in a medical school, a community hospital, an office building, an industrial plant, or a specially constructed facility. Wherever health care practitioners pool their professional financial resources in the care of individual patients, there is group practice in the midst of them. These comments were shared at a joint session of the Medical Care, Public Health Nursing, and Statistical Sections of the American Public Health Association annual meeting in St. Louis, Missouri, October 31, 1950. They were published in the December 1950 issue of the American Journal of Public Health *many years before the term "Health Maintenance Organization" was developed to designate group payment for group practice.*

Patterns and Problems of Group Medical Practice

There has been a radical revolution in medical science, which is now being followed by a gradual evolution in medical practice. Group medical service is being developed to coordinate the specialized knowledge and skill of individual practitioners, and to utilize effectively the public's investment in diagnostic and treatment facilities, including hospitals.

In discussing the patterns and problems of group medical practice, the following statements about medical care are presented as objectives concerning which there can be no dispute, or self-evident facts which do not require proof in this essay.

1. Comprehensive medical service includes prevention, diagnosis, treatment, case finding, rehabilitation, and health education.

2. Good medical care should be coordinated, continuous, and related to the entire personality and the individual's environment.

3. Education and research are closely related to service and cannot be sharply segregated.

4. Medical practitioners can accomplish better results by working *with* each other than *against* each other.

5. Medical care can be produced and distributed most effectively when physicians and patients are free to perform and receive services with a minimum of concern about financial costs.

6. Health practitioners and patients strive more or less consciously toward these ends in all medical service programs.

Group Medical Practice is a program for prevention, diagnosis, and treatment, the essential characteristic of which is a *common interest by a number of physicians in the care of individual patients.* The doctors share their knowledge and skill in determining and providing the necessary services. Observable features of group practice include: specialized professional qualifications of the practitioners; contiguity of professional offices with availability for regular and frequent consultations concerning individual patients; joint use of supplementary services; some joint ownership of equipment, apparatus, or buildings; cooperative, rather than competitive division of total income among the group.

Origins of Group Medical Practice

Group practice is a process, rather than a form of organization. The central theme—a common interest in the patient—is always present. But the variations are numerous. Some group practice may be *intermittent*, rather than continuous, as in the exchange of opinion during ward-rounds in a hospital. Some group practice may be *part-time*, rather than full-time, as in the sessions attended in a hospital outpatient department, or office appointments at a clinic serving prepayment contract patients. Some group practice is for *diagnosis* only, with treatment procedures becoming the responsibility of individual doctors. Some group practice is limited to *special groups*, such as contract patients, rather than the general public. Some group practice is limited to *referred cases* with no acceptance of patients who do not have a personal physician. Some group practice is limited to economic classes, such as persons of *moderate means* or those unable to pay current established fees.

The evolution of group practice was inevitable. The *development of specialization* in medical knowledge and skill has forced a degree of coordination in medical practice. This trend is similar to that which occurred in private business when artisans began to specialize in detailed processes of building construction, the manufacture of clothes, or the preparation of food. As medical knowledge deepens in specific areas, it must be shared through conference and observation; otherwise, its values are not effectively utilized in prevention, diagnosis, and treatment. Medical service has become characterized by an *increasing reliance upon capital investment* for adequate diagnosis and treatment. Illustrations are X-ray apparatus, laboratory equipment, operating rooms, and complete hospitals for bed cases. Even if one doctor could finance the purchase of such plant and equipment, he could not personally perform each professional or technical service. He would need to rely upon subordinate or coordinate practitioners for most of the work, who, in turn, would be required to coordinate their services by conferences, records, and reports.

Specialization in knowledge and skill and the use of capital investment in medical practice are *causes*, not *results*, of group practice. The
scientific and economic aspects of present-day health service make it
necessary that the various phases of diagnosis and treatment be coordinated. *The general hospital is the natural site for the greatest development
of group practice in America.* The medical specialists are already spending
a great deal of time at hospitals in the care of patients who need bed
care during a portion of their diagnosis and treatment. The hospitals
contain the greatest portion of the specialized equipment for diagnosis
and treatment, together with a full-time staff trained to use the facilities
under medical supervision.

There has been a traditional Chinese Wall between services to horizontal and vertical patients in hospitals. But the gates were opened
when private practitioners found it more convenient to serve their
nonpaying ambulatory patients at the hospital where publicly provided
apparatus could be used without a rental charge to the doctor, and
where nurses and medical students were available to assist the private
physicians. The individual doctors are now finding it increasingly convenient to use hospital facilities for the consultations and treatments
for paying cases.

Patterns of Group Practice

The patterns of group practice in the United States may be classified
by several standards, such as degree of full-time participation, degree
of hospital affiliation, scope of health services offered, groups eligible
for service, or other bases. The following listing emphasizes the administrative characteristics of various forms of group practice. It does
not include the hospital outpatient departments conducted for the
"worthy poor."

Private group clinics. This form of group medicine includes a number of individual practitioners representing several specialties, who work
together in adjacent offices, most of them on a full-time basis. They
usually rely upon local hospitals for the bed care of their patients and
for provision of the more unusual types of scientific apparatus and
equipment; but they may own and operate radiological and pathological laboratories and may perform minor operations at the central offices. They are in economic competition with other doctors, but not
with each other.

The headquarters may be in office buildings or separate structures
which are owned or rented. The doctors are usually organized in part-

nerships, but corporations may be established for the ownership of property and the employment of the doctors. Ordinarily, the clinics are open to the general public for all types of service, but a certain number of cases are referred by other doctors. They may have special contracts with insured patients, but most groups rely upon such revenue only to a limited degree.

Private clinics tend to be located in the smaller cities, and the medical personnel ranges from 3 to 300 individuals. The largest number have been organized west of the Mississippi River, in part through the influence of the Mayo Clinic at Rochester, Minn. The number of such groups is variously estimated at from 300 to 500, depending on the standards used for the listing.

This form of group practice represents the pattern most easily applied to present-day medicine by a group of physicians desiring to coordinate their efforts in the prevention, diagnosis, and treatment of disease and in the study and development of a positive health program. Some of the private clinics established to serve individual patients have relied greatly upon prepayment contracts with groups of employees and their dependents or with employers for the care of industrial compensation cases. An example of this type of clinic is the Ross-Loos Medical Group in Los Angeles, organized in 1929. It now includes 115 physicians and serves about 110,000 people on an insurance contract basis, as well as the general public. Hospital care is obtained in local institutions.

Full-time hospital staffs. The outstanding example of this type of group practice is the Ford Hospital, established in 1915 at Detroit, Mich. Other significant examples are the Cleveland Clinic and Hospital, the Geisinger Hospital at Danville, Pa., the Guthrie Clinic and Robert Packer Hospital at Sayre, Pa., the Hitchcock Memorial Hospital, Hanover, N. H., the Underwood Hospital, Woodbury, N. J., and the Trinity Hospital, Little Rock, Ark.

These groups merge the outpatient and inpatient professional services at the hospital; the physicians are engaged on a full-time basis for annual salaries; the institution is open to the general public for both general and specialized care and for referred and walk-in patients. An exception is the Pratt Diagnostic Clinic and New England Medical Center Hospital, Boston, which are limited almost exclusively to cases referred by other physicians.

This form of full-time closed staff has seldom developed (if ever) from a community general hospital with an attending and courtesy staff. Usually, the institutions have established closed staffs at the time of their organization. In some cases, a private clinic has obtained control of an existing hospital or has constructed bed facilities for its own use. Combined institutions with full-time closed staffs have seldom been the recipients of city-wide philanthropy. But a number control endowment funds provided by an original donor or accrued from the net earnings of the private medical practice.

These organizations may accept insurance patients on the same basis as other practitioners and hospitals, but typically they do not rely upon group prepayment for their financial support.

In this group may be included the full-time medical faculty of the University of Chicago Clinics which accept diagnostic and treatment cases from all income levels in the general public, and which utilize all patients as teaching material when they are suitable for the purpose.

Medical groups organized for insured or other special groups. Within the past three decades a number of clinics have been established to serve special groups of the general public. These include the full-time staffs of industrial plants, such as the Endicott-Johnson Company and the many private clinics in the Pacific Coast States which have contracts with employed firms to serve their employees and dependents.

More significant for the future are the groups established in connection with consumers who have provided capital facilities on a cooperative basis with small contributions from each member eligible to medical service benefits. Examples are the Elk City Hospital in Oklahoma, the Labor Health Institute in St. Louis, and the Group Health Cooperatives in Seattle and the District of Columbia. The clinics typically accept patients from the general public, and some of the practitioners are engaged on a part-time basis for service at the clinic. But the final objective in most instances is the development of a full-time staff devoted to a program of constructive health service on a prepayment basis.

The giant in this category of group practice is the Health Insurance Plan of Greater New York, which has aided in the establishment of 30 medical groups, with a total of 900 physicians, to serve the now 250,000 participants in a comprehensive prepayment program for prevention, diagnosis, treatment, and health education. This organization began services to patients in 1947, and was aided in its establishment by grants from several foundations. H. I. P. is one of the few organizations which began with a three-dimensional program, namely: full-time group practice by doctors; group prepayment for entire families; comprehensive service in the home, office, and hospital. Most other organizations established either group practice or group prepayment independently of each other, and usually limited the service to specialty work or the coverage to catastrophic illnesses.

Part-time medical groups. These groups are usually limited by the character of service provided or the method in which cases are accepted. Examples are the Mt. Sinai Diagnostic Clinic in New York for referred patients of moderate means; the Vanderbilt Clinic in New York for diagnosis and treatment of patients of limited incomes; the Benjamin Franklin Clinic of the Pennsylvania Hospital in Philadelphia for flat rate diagnostic service to referred patients of any income level; the Private Out-Patient Service of the Johns Hopkins Hospital, Baltimore; the Boston Dispensary which provides home care, as well as office service.

The part-time clinics have not grown rapidly in number, although some have increased their volume of service greatly, as the public has become aware of the available benefits. As a general rule, "reference" clinics have relied upon cases referred by doctors outside the immediate private practice trading area. This form of organization tends to become a general service available to walk-in patients, or to remain a limited activity for the convenience of the member physicians rather than the general profession and population. Diagnosis and treatment are inseparable in the patient's mind, and attempts to maintain a division are not approved or accepted by the general public.

Private ambulatory service. The most prevalent, but least spectacular, group practice is the intermittent or regular use by individual doctors of hospital personnel and facilities in diagnostic service for private patients. This may take the form of reference of a patient to the hospital for X-ray films, examination, or treatment, for laboratory examination, or for conference with various medical specialists. The doctor may utilize hospital consulting rooms on a regular or intermittent basis for conferences with his patients and the various members of the hospital staff.

This trend represents "group practice *a la carte.*" The solo doctor may carry it *as far as* he wishes, and *when* he wishes. But the practice is growing rapidly. In total volume this work probably exceeds that of organized group practice by full-time and part-time clinics throughout the country.

Some physicians have viewed this trend with alarm, as placing the hospital in the practice of medicine, and making the solo doctor dependent on hospital personnel and facilities for the conduct of his practice. But service to private ambulatory patients may be more accurately regarded as a protector of individual practice, the absence of which would require direct hospital control over much diagnostic and treatment service. The alternative would be for the solo doctor to continue hand-bag medicine without regular contacts with specialized knowledge, skill, and facilities. Moreover, the regular contacts by general practitioners with hospitals may lead to appropriate staff appointments for such physicians and their integration with formal group practice which may develop at such institutions.

Physicians should be guided by enlightened self-interest in their decisions to participate in group medical practice. The "fate worse than debt" for the physician is the loss of self-determination in the practice of his profession. Statistics indicate that, on the average, physicians fare better financially under group practice than individual practice. But specific individuals (often the ones with the administrative genius to organize a group) might earn more income "on their own," and also be free from the trials of holding a medical group together. *Leadership is the missing link in the growth of group practice, for those best able to organize a group often have the least financial incentive to do so.*

Problems of Group Practice

The following list of problems facing the establishment and continuance of group medical practice does not cover all opportunities and difficulties which must be faced, but they are submitted as representatives of some of those which will be faced at one time or another:

1. *Motivation.* A clinic may be established for any of a variety of reasons, such as: the improvement of quality of medical care; the lowering of costs to patients; the increasing of income to physicians; the stabilization of working conditions for doctors; the training of subsidiary personnel; a demonstration of the advantages of coordinated practice; the freeing of physicians from direct concern about economic problems. In the writer's opinion, *the sustaining motivation for physicians must be their personal self-interest, not social reform or demonstrations in medical economics, or even the avoidance of socialized medicine.*

Self-interest cannot be measured exclusively in terms of current income or future estate. More important is the opportunity for personal and professional self-realization. Group practice must expand rather than contract the doctor's opportunity to work as an individual and a professional man. The economic security of group practice must be accompanied by personal freedom to care for patients in accord with their needs, and to practice medicine at the highest attainable level of quality.

Much discussion of group practice has assumed that it is a form of revolution in the field of health service. From a logical point of view, a medical group is no more revolutionary than a baseball team. Each member has his position to play, and effectiveness depends upon team work rather than star performance. In the long run, group practice must reward individual doctors more adequately than does individual practice.

2. *Provision of working capital.* Group practice involves less per-capita investment by medical practitioners than does a group of individual private offices. The borrowing power of a partnership is enhanced by the demonstration of willingness to cooperate in professional activity. Vendors of scientific apparatus and equipment are typically more willing to extend credit to a group of physicians than to individual doctors. A group of physicians who have determined to carry on group practice seldom face difficulties in obtaining necessary working capital. Moreover, they can begin with partial facilities and arrange for temporary use of special apparatus on a rental or fee basis from other organizations.

3. *Selection of site.* There is no one best location for a private clinic, geographically or as to type of building structure. Downtown offices, separate suburban buildings, portions of a hospital plant—all have advantages and limitations. Other things being equal, a medical group should not be too far away from the patients to be served or the related facilities (such as hospitals) which are utilized from time to time. But the public will soon discover the source of good service.

4. *Scope of service.* Medical groups should be prepared to deal with all types of illness and any member of the population. If the group does not include the specialized knowledge and skill for certain treatment, arrangements should be established for other physicians and institutions to furnish necessary care. As a general rule, a clinic should direct patients to proper medical service, rather than merely refuse to accept certain categories of illnesses or of the population.

The number and specialties within the medical group are influenced by a variety of factors such as size of the community, available supplementary facilities, and the prospective amount of referred work as contrasted with care of minor ailments. An important factor is the degree to which a medical group utilizes subordinate personnel for routine diagnostic or treatment procedures, as well as personal contacts with patients.

5. *Fees to be charged.* A medical group should not be a "cut rate" organization, but should be able to offer a patient (or group of patients) more for his money than an equal number of competing practitioners. It is the total cost, rather than the detailed charges, which interests the prospective or actual patient. Composite fees established in advance give a sense of security and gratitude to the patient. He often will pay in full because of the certainty as to the amount. Medical groups are particularly equipped to establish composite fees for a variety of different services, since the total income accrues to all practitioners.

6. *Distribution of income.* Most defunct clinics have prospered financially, as far as total income is concerned, up to the point of dissolution. Without exception, their greatest difficulty was the determination of each physician's share in the net earnings of the group. A medical group cannot distribute net earnings to physicians solely on the basis of each one's volume of service.

Variables to be recognized in establishing a doctor's share in the net income of group practice include the following: degree of administrative responsibility; amount of capital investment; length of service with the group; demonstrable popularity with old patients; demonstrable "pulling power" with new patients; contribution to quality of service through research or teaching ability; interest in health conservation and health education; relative scarcity of his special knowledge or skill; and ability to perform an unusual volume of high quality service.

7. *Relations with individual practitioners.* A medical group is both a supplement and a competitor of the practice of individual doctors. Even referral groups are a potential threat to the economic security of nonmember physicians. Competition based on quality, rather than price, will ultimately win the respect of many individual doctors. The maintenance of cordial professional and personal relations with nongroup physicians requires considerable effort and attention.

8. *Relations with hospitals.* These problems are continuous for medical groups and often very difficult. Under ordinary circumstances, use of a voluntary hospital is preferred to the purchase and management of a proprietary institution. In the long run, it is more rewarding to make peace with the local medical profession concerning use of an existing hospital than to run the risk of excessive facilities by establishment of a new institution.

9. *Use of subsidiary personnel.* The medical supervision possible in a clinic permits nurses and other technically trained employees to perform many procedures which otherwise consume the time of a physician. This applies particularly to the use of nurses in response to house calls and the performance of follow-up procedures prescribed by a physician.

It is desirable that a nurse should not "practice medicine." But it is also important that a doctor should be freed from the necessity of performing nursing procedures.

Group practice should permit specialists to use their knowledge and skill to the greatest degree. General practitioners and nonmedical personnel should be colleagues rather than competitors.

10. *Varied administrative problems.* Group medical practice faces many administrative problems in its development and growth. Some of them are:

a. Care of patients during personal absences;

b. Need for intensive service to cases requiring special study;

c. Old age and retirement allowances;

d. Full-time use of young physicians;

e. "Tapering-off" of services by older physicians;

f. Attention to health education;

g. Skillful and humane handling of malingerers;

h. Attention to psychological factors in treatment and recovery;

i. Responsibility for home calls and night service;

j. Recognition of unusual knowledge or skill;

k. Scheduling the use of apparatus and equipment;

l. Informal consultations in diagnosis or treatment;

m. Authoritative contacts with regulatory bodies;

n. Interpretation of services to the general public;

o. Sub-contracting with prepayment organizations, particularly for home and office calls which involve a substantial degree of "moral hazard";

p. Periodic appraisal of quality of service;

q. Study of medical records; and

r. Statistical analysis of services performed and results achieved.

Conclusions

1. The development of group medical practice will be dependent upon the degree to which doctors consider such activities as favorable to their immediate and long-run self-interest. Opportunity for unfettered professional service is a greater factor than size of total income.

2. Doctors with a genius for business organization are also usually successful private practitioners. The main administrative need in group practice is an attitude of common concern for the patient's recovery and health maintenance. This is more important than brilliance in the field of management, or unusual scientific knowledge and skill. In group practice the whole is greater than the sum of its parts.

3. Courage and determination are more important than plant and equipment or working capital. The public stands ready to provide working capital for responsible medical groups by one of three processes:

a. Contributions by patients who expect to be served, such as members of a cooperative or insurance organization;

b. Private loans from commercial banks or vendors of medical equipment; and

c. Offers of the use of public facilities in hospitals or health agencies.

4. An important area for the development of medical group practice is the gradual transformation of hospital outpatient departments from limited service for the "worthy poor" to general service to the entire public.

5. "Restrictive" group practice will probably not become a significant phase of medical service in the United States. This prediction applies particularly to diagnostic or referral clinics, as well as medical groups limited to service to industrial firms or single insurance corporations.

6. The public does not distinguish between functions of diagnosis and treatment and wishes to receive complete medical care from the same medical organization.

7. Group medical practice is a way of life and an attitude toward health service, not merely an administrative device to increase quality, reduce costs, or to stabilize medical income.

8. Group medical practice is a process of evolution which is developing gradually. It is following upon a series of "revolutions" in medical science. Specialized knowledge and skill in the field of medicine require the use of group practice in their application to prevention, diagnosis, and treatment. But a cultural lag still remains between what is *known*, and what is *being done* about it.

Obstetrical services require well-trained personnel and specialized facilities, which must be utilized to the optimum if quality is to be maintained and costs controlled. A study by Marvin D. Roth and me, both on the staff of the Health and Hospital Council of Southern New York, showed that many hospitals were serving surprisingly small numbers of obstetrical cases per year. We recommended that obstetrical care in the New York area be concentrated in a relatively few institutions. This policy would release much space for ambulatory care and general surgical and medical service. The report was published in the December 16, 1966 issue of Hospitals, *journal of the American Hospital Association.*

Need Every Hospital Offer an Obstetric Service?

A 69-bed hospital in southern New York recently faced the following problem: Its 13 obstetric beds averaged 4 obstetric patients a day while its 56 medical-surgical beds averaged 50 patients per day. The obstetric beds were being utilized at one-third of capacity while the medical-surgical beds were being used at 90 percent of capacity.

The administrator attempted to solve this problem by converting five maternity beds to medical-surgical use and also by converting one nursery to an area housing five additional medical-surgical beds. Before implementing this decision, however, he analyzed his daily obstetric census and found that on only seven days during the entire year were there more than eight maternity patients in the hospital. He concluded, therefore, that he need operate only eight obstetric beds. On the few days during the year when the maternity unit was overcrowded, peak loads could be handled by early discharge of a patient, the use of a labor room for a brief period of time, or by placing patients in the solarium on the obstetric floor.

This problem is not uncommon. More than 20 hospitals in southern New York face the same problem; possibly several thousand others across the country do also. In fact, it is estimated that close to half the hospitals in the country operating maternity departments have an average census of five or fewer maternity patients a day.

Question to Answer

The administrator's decision to reduce the number of maternity beds and use them for medical-surgical patients was based upon the assumption that the hospital should maintain an obstetric service. He might well have asked the following question: Should this hospital maintain an obstetric service?

The individual hospital cannot resolve this problem alone. The solution should be developed from a community-wide point of view, preferably by an areawide planning agency, with the number and types of other hospitals serving the area taken into consideration.

Duplication of Facilities

The overabundance of maternity and newborn facilities results from the interplay of many factors. During the post-World War II period, the number of births in the nation increased from less than 2.9 million in 1946 to a peak of 4.3 million in 1957 and the number of newborn accommodations increased from 85,000 to 105,000 bassinets. However, the declining number of births in recent years—4.1 million babies were born in 1964—combined with a 50 percent reduction in length of stay for maternity patients (from 9 days in 1946 to 4.5 days in 1964) has resulted in a large number of vacant maternity beds. In fact, the average daily maternity census for all hospitals in the United States declined from 53,000 in 1946 to 45,000 last year. There were 60,000 vacant maternity beds on an average day last year.

These vacant maternity beds can be used for other services. Although the occupancy rate for all hospitals in the nation has ranged from 80 to 85 percent in the last two decades, the utilization of obstetric facilities has declined from approximately 62 percent in 1946 to less than 45 percent last year.

The probability is very small that all of the 105,000 maternity beds in this country will be required in the near future. This can be predicted safely by reviewing the history of obstetric practice. Originally, all babies were born at home. As recently as 1942, one baby out of every three was still born at home. Last year, about two percent of all babies were born at home. The transfer of obstetric care from the home to the hospital occurred gradually throughout the country.

However, an increased use of obstetric facilities will no longer occur merely by transferring the place of birth from the home to the hospital. Additional facilities will be required only in those rapidly growing parts of the country where there is still a sizable increase in the number of births. This situation creates the possibility of utilizing vacant obstetric facilities in many institutions for other types of professional care for which there is a present need.

Council Study Findings

Recently the Hospital Review and Planning Council of Southern New York conducted a special study of obstetric facilities in its region with a view to developing guidelines and recommendations for their effective use and future planning. The inquiry was concerned with both quality of care and efficiency of individual obstetric departments. Among the council's major findings were the following:

1. *Obstetrical facilities in southern New York are ineffectively located and utilized.* There is an oversupply in some areas and inadequate provision in others. There are many small maternity units that are uneconomical and inefficient to operate. They are unable to provide high quality care during a period of rising costs and declining occupancy.

This evaluation of obstetric facilities and utilization was conducted in terms of community needs and planning. There was no attempt to establish standards of obstetric practice, but the suggested guidelines are consistent with recommendations of national professional bodies, and also with the public interest reflected in existing legislation and health codes related to maternity and infant care.

2. *Large-scale operation requires relatively fewer nursing personnel, who are already in short supply.* The most important factor is compliance with minimum staffing requirements established by state and local health codes.

The New York City health code requires the services of at least 11 registered nurses each day regardless of the number of obstetric patients. These 11 nurses are sufficient to staff a maternity department when the average census ranges from one to seven mothers. However, when the average census exceeds seven, additional nursing personnel are required. A maternity unit with 28 mothers, for instance, requires 24 nursing personnel per day; twice as many are required to staff a unit with a census four times as great. Also, of the 24 nursing personnel required for the larger census, only 15 need to be registered nurses; the other 9 could be aides or practical nurses.

The data indicate that the ratio of the minimum number of nurses required per mother declines as the average daily maternity census increases. But the rate of change in this ratio starts to decrease after a level of 28 mothers per day is reached. Do these lower ratios of nursing personnel per patient mean that the larger units provide a lower quality of service? Not at all. Smaller units frequently must employ more obstetric nurses than are necessary to serve their patients, or they will violate provisions of the local health code by permitting obstetric nurses to work elsewhere in the hospital during periods of reduced activity in the maternity department.

3. *Larger obstetrical units in southern New York experience higher annual occupancy rates than smaller units.* The obstetric beds in 115 hospitals reporting less than 2,000 live births each during 1964, for example, were occupied at only 54 percent of capacity. For the 38 hospitals with more than 2,000 births in 1964, the average was 71 percent. The explanation lies partly in the fact that proportionally fewer vacant beds have to be held in readiness in the larger obstetric units.

4. *Cost per maternity delivery tends to vary inversely with the volume of obstetric service.* To assure comparability, the 1964 financial experience of 38 obstetric departments in New York City was examined. It was found that the direct costs of the delivery rooms, as recorded in the accounts of each institution, were proportionally lower in the larger programs than in the smaller. The average direct cost per delivery was $47, for example, for the 18 hospitals reporting less than 2,000 births during the year. For 20 larger programs, the average was $38 per delivery. This finding is especially significant because the larger programs included most of the hospitals conducting educational programs and to which many difficult cases are referred for specialized services.

5. *Quality of obstetric care tends to be higher when the volume of obstetric services increases.* The larger programs are able to attract better trained and more qualified professional staff and to justify investment in expensive equipment and facilities. These programs also provide a basis for teaching programs for resident physicians, interns, and professional nurses. The larger units also permit layout and design for effective protection of obstetric and other patients.

6. *The Council concluded that the southern New York region would be better served by the operation of fewer but larger obstetric programs.* There are 153 obstetric units in southern New York, ranging in bed capacity from 2 to 134 beds and in number of annual live births from less than 100 to more than 6,500 per institution. The 5,200 obstetrical beds were utilized at 62 percent of capacity during 1964, with an average of 2,000 vacant beds per day. A total of 110 obstetrical units with an average of 40 beds each could have accommodated the 260,000 maternity admissions—if they had been operating at 75 percent of capacity with an

average stay of five days. This would be possible because most parts of the New York area have large population concentrations.

Major Council Recommendations

Accordingly, the council made the following recommendations:

In densely populated areas, only hospitals with a volume of 2,000 or more births per year should operate maternity departments. The various analyses relating births to staffing patterns, costs, and utilization indicated a significant break point was attained in a unit with 2,000 or more live births per year. A unit with this volume of activity requires 36 to 40 beds. Also, since staffing is related both to number of beds and number of nurses' stations, these beds should be on one nurses' station. This volume of service would apply only to the more densely populated urban areas of the country. It will still be necessary for hospitals in the sparsely settled rural areas to operate maternity departments even though they have far less than 2,000 births per year.

Obstetric and newborn infant care should be rendered only at general hospitals large enough to provide necessary ancillary services. Many specialized maternity hospitals have not been able to provide the diagnostic and treatment services required for the care of mothers and newborn infants in emergencies and complicated cases. An effective program requires the availability of personnel and equipment to give clinical and pathological tests, X-ray examinations and treatments, special care of the newborn infants, psychiatric services, and social service to patients and families that need support and guidance in solving their problems. It is not essential that every general hospital conduct an obstetric service, but it is important that every obstetric service be conducted at a general hospital that is large enough to assure comprehensive health service.

Every effort should be made to achieve flexibility in the use of maternity facilities, within the framework of existing regulations. Special attention should be given to alternate use of obstetric beds during periods of low occupancy. Professional judgment indicates that admission of selected gynecologic patients to obstetric bed facilities, under controlled conditions, does not jeopardize the quality of service. In several communities—Chicago, Pittsburgh, northern New Jersey—special studies and experimentation have supported medical opinion in this regard.

Another example of flexible use of bed facilities is the establishment of "swing" units, which are available for obstetric and other patients, and which include movable partitions, separate call systems, and nurses' stations. Swing units may be designed at slight extra cost when new construction is undertaken. Mention should be made of the advantage of using total obstetric accommodations for all maternity cases and newborn infants, regardless of their financial sponsorship or professional relations with attending staff. Separate units for ward or private patients create the same problems as small obstetric units when the patient census varies from time to time.

Hospital obstetric programs should include ambulatory care (prenatal and postnatal) to assure continuity of service to maternity patients and newborn infants. Hospitalization of an obstetric patient normally requires only four to six days at time of delivery, but adequate care involves professional supervision and advice for several months before and after. This care should include initial valuation of the patient's medical, nursing, and social service needs. Facilities for emergency treatment should also be available. Such a program can be offered most effectively at a general hospital providing similar services for other ambulatory patients.

Pediatric and premature infant services should be available and accessible to all maternity departments. A qualified pediatrician should be available to assume responsibility for the care of newborn infants from the initial physical examination until the child is discharged from the hospital. This does not mean that every hospital serving obstetric patients should also maintain an organized service for pediatric patients. But it is essential that the professional care of newborn infants be supervised by physicians who are qualified in this field. Facilities for the care of premature infants are not essential at every hospital, but such service should be readily available at properly staffed premature centers to which infants may be transferred when necessary.

Coordination among hospitals in accepting maternity admissions would result in great convenience and savings for a community. Coordination offers special values when the consolidation of smaller programs or construction of larger units is not feasible. This would require the extension of staff privileges to all qualified obstetricians at institutions located in the same community. The practice would tend to reduce the daily fluctuation of occupancy at individual hospitals. When one institution is crowded and another has empty beds, a physician should be able to use any available hospital bed without disrupting the physician-patient relationship. Each staff appointment should entail an equitable contribution by the obstetrician to community service and to care of patients with limited financial resources.

Conclusion

A coordinated program of concentrating obstetric care in fewer institutions would be of great value to the entire population of a multi-hospital community. It would (1) provide better use of existing capital investment; (2) permit some institutions to utilize much needed bed capacity for services to medical and surgical patients; (3) raise the standards of obstetric care at the institutions that continue their programs; and (4) improve the quality of health service for other patients at the hospitals that transfer their obstetric services to other institutions. An areawide planning agency has both a challenge and an opportunity to persuade hospitals to cooperate in the provision of adequate obstetric care for the communities they serve.

Part Two

Group Payment for Health Care

Comment

C. Rufus Rorem is an extremely practical visionary. Is he too practical, too visionary? I've never been able to make up my mind about such questions but always find his combination of "here and now" objectives and long-range perspective most useful in addressing health problems. This small self-selected sampling of his writings provides a new opportunity to speculate about Dr. Rorem's unique way of dealing with immediate problems in a secure "futures" framework.

From 1932 to 1947 (when I first met him), group payment for health care was the central but not exclusive focus of his professional life and the chief beneficiary of his unique analytical skills. The legacy of this period is not only a series of brilliant essays that can be read and reread with continuing benefit but also a novel social institution, Blue Cross.

The Blue Cross system continues to struggle with long-range problems within the framework delineated by Dr. Rorem. Anyone interested in the future directions of Blue Cross will gain as much insight from reviewing Dr. Rorem's papers as from studying current pronouncements or decisions of Blue Cross executives.

The essays concerning group payment for health care selected by Dr. Rorem for inclusion in this collection may stimulate some readers to search well-stocked libraries for the essays that were excluded. Included here are his first published paper on group payment, a consultant report to the American Hospital Association on progress in forming hospital service plans up to 1934, his last major presentation as a Blue Cross official, and other papers written during this phase of his career. There are also two papers written after he turned over the Blue Cross reins in 1947; these provide insights about group payment through national government and commercial insurance, supplementing the focus on community-based programs.

In the first paper (1932), Dr. Rorem classifies the many forms of group payment for medical care in the United States. He notes that there is a wide range of programs, but very few participating policyholders or providers. In describing and classifying the national experiments that had sprouted in all parts of the country, Dr. Rorem helps to define many of the issues that have occupied students and practitioners in the field during the past half century. Fifty years ago, hospitalization plans were spreading rapidly, but there was no prototype of Blue Cross. A year later, but before E. A. van Steenwyck devised the Blue Cross symbol in Minnesota, Dr. Rorem addressed the benefits of such arrangements for hospitals and the public and the specific tasks involved in planning and managing group hospitalization plans.

Though readers can test their analytic skills by trying to identify points where Dr. Rorem went wrong, they will not be able to identify many key issues that he overlooked. Dr. Rorem was always more interested in getting something done than in getting something perfect, but he never worked within a narrow perspective.

In the years that followed, there was much debate about compulsory versus voluntary health insurance; Dr. Rorem pushed voluntary health insurance forward. He thought it more productive to debate with those who opposed compulsory insurance than with those who viewed it as a precondition for improved health services. This collection includes a "debate" with Morris Fishbein, but not with those who condemned voluntary group payment as "a new and massive bulwark for the organizational status quo." To the best of my knowledge, Dr. Rorem felt that the debate about which must come first, group payment or group practice, was either sterile or counterproductive. He never supported those who felt that group payment and group practice had to be linked from the beginning, but I don't think he ever doubted that they would ultimately be conjoined.

His presentation about Blue Cross at the U.S. Congress just before he decided to leave the field of health services financing to return to his first passion—the provision of health services—is instructive for his views of the issues facing the then well-established Blue Cross system and of the role the federal government could play. As always, his suggestions were extremely practical; all have now been incorporated in the law and in administrative regulations.

His 1953 paper on commercial insurance suggests standards comparable to the standards he had developed for Blue Cross two decades earlier. Adoption of these standards today would encourage health marketplace competition. While these standards have never been formally adopted, the leadership of the commercial insurance industry has made substantial progress on four of the seven directions set forth; the others are being considered but are thought to require legislation providing an antitrust exemption. If such legislation were adopted today, the practicality of Dr. Rorem's suggestions could be tested. In 1953, lack of trust between the companies seemed to be a greater obstacle than fear of antitrust litigation. Has this really changed?

The review of developments in England in 1947 reveals a strong preference for voluntary leadership and initiative in attacking problems that society must address. His view of the potential public service role of voluntary institutions is a challenge to physicians and hospitals to provide the leadership necessary to avoid either government-controlled health insurance or a complete system of state medicine.

Dr. Rorem's papers are being published at a time when the federal government is assigning greater value to free competition in the health market than to assurance of equity in health care. These papers should encourage all of us in the health field to face up to our opportunities for public service. They remind us of all that an energetic, clear thinking, pragmatic individual can accomplish.

Robert M. Sigmond

Health care insurance coverage in the early 1930s was very thinly spread. There were many varieties of plans, but the total participation was less than one percent of the population. For the most part, programs were sponsored by employers operating in areas where medical facilities were scarce, such as lumber camps, mines, western railroads, and temporary construction projects. Some fraternal organizations employed "lodge doctors" to provide limited services to members. Total membership accelerated with the establishment of hospital service plans and contract practice by groups of physicians. The next selection, originally published in the June 1932 issue of the Bulletin *of the American Hospital Association, describes the situation before the advent of Group Hospitalization (later known as Blue Cross) and other community plans providing comprehensive health care.*

Sickness Insurance in the United States

The people of the United States spend, on the average, about twenty-five or thirty dollars per year for medical care. But the costs of medical care are not equally distributed among the population. Moreover, the need for medical care is not restricted to those able to pay for it. The costs of caring for a single illness may vary from five dollars to one thousand dollars or more.

The Unevenness of the Burden

Only a fraction of any group of the population is afflicted with severe illness during the year. But on some persons the financial burden falls heavily. Extensive studies by the United States Bureau of Labor Statistics and recently by the Committee on the Costs of Medical Care show that more than half of the total family expenditure for the year for general sickness falls upon less than 15 per cent of the families.

The total cost of medical care may be predicted and estimated in advance for a group of people, but not for an individual member of the group. The cost of sickness cannot be budgeted by an individual with the same certainty with which he can plan his expenditures for rent, light, food, clothing, automobiles, radios, etc. For, even though the individual budgets a reasonable amount, say one hundred dollars per year for medical care, he has no assurance that he will not incur an expense of three or four hundred dollars. Moreover, accidents during the following year, or even within the same year, may require additional expenditures of equal amounts.

Costs of sickness are compulsory, and must be met by the patient, the public, or the physician. A group of people can do what the individual cannot do, namely, budget the costs of their medical care. By "group payment" for the services which individuals in the group will require, numbers of people can frequently assure themselves of medical care at costs which are within their ability to pay. There are in the United States several types of medical organizations which apply the principle of "group payment" for the costs of medical care. These procedures may be referred to as sickness insurance, although most of the arrangements are not classified as insurance contracts by the respective states.

The Financial Risks of Illness

Two types of financial risk result from illness—(a) the loss of money income, (b) the costs of medical care. Some life insurance companies, and the various casualty and accident companies, provide a monetary benefit during a period of unemployment resulting from an accident or from a disability caused by sickness. Usually the amount of benefit is based upon the premium paid by the policyholder or upon the salary or income which was received up to the time of the disability. As a rule these companies do not provide medical care, nor do they guarantee to reimburse the insured persons for the costs of medical care. The rates for such protection are relatively high and are carried by people in the upper middle classes, or the well-to-do. Some of the casualty and indemnity associations also write group insurance against loss of money income by individuals during periods of accident or illness. There are also sick-benefit clubs organized by trade unions or by lodges which provide monetary benefits during periods of illness or accident to their members. In some instances these benefits also include a certain amount of medical care from a lodge doctor. On the whole, however, the monetary benefit is very limited and the quality of the service exceedingly poor.

Old-line life insurance companies have not found the sale of individual insurance policies for the costs of medical care to be profitable. The more sickly tend to insure, particularly where monetary benefits are granted during the period of illness. None of the large insurance companies provides medical care directly to its policyholders. Insurance against the costs of medical care has not been developed through the usual life or casualty insurance procedures. There are, however, several types of agreement by which groups of individuals have voluntarily applied the insurance principle, that is, "group payment," in the payment for medical or hospital care, or both. It is with such agreements that this paper is primarily concerned. Some of the agreements apply to hospital services exclusively, and some to physicians' services exclusively, whereas others deal with complete medical care.

Industrial Medical Service

A survey by the National Tuberculosis Association revealed that approximately four hundred different business enterprises have established more or less complete medical services for their employees. No two plans are identical as to method of financing or as to scope of the services made available to the employees.

The industrial medical services had their origin in the mining, lumber, and railroad industries, when employees of this type of enterprise were faced with difficulty in obtaining the services of local physicians. As a consequence the employer often engaged the full-time or part-time services of one or more physicians on behalf of his employees. The difficulties of transportation which originally prompted the industrial medical services in the railroad, mining, and lumbering industries have in part disappeared. But the medical services have been continued in these industries, as well as in large industrial organizations. More recently less hazardous enterprises, such as department stores, warehouses, and printing establishments, have instituted medical services for their employees.

The principle underlying the provision of industrial medical services, particularly in those instances where the employer has borne a large share of the burden, has been the desire to establish and maintain an effective working force. In many instances the medical services began as physical examinations requisite to employment; in other cases the medical examination was the basis for assignment to particular types of activity within the plant. In any event, industrial medical service appears to be a permanent part of the business organization of this country, and approximately two million workers are estimated to receive more or less complete industrial medical service.

The medical care referred to as industrial medical service is not to be confused with the services financed and provided under the Workmen's Compensation Insurance agreements in the various states. Industrial medical facilities and personnel may, of course, be used to render care for compensable accident cases.

Employee Contributions

In Oregon and Washington, about ten years ago, private medical insurance companies were formed to make contracts with employers to provide services for accidents which are compensable under the Workmen's Compensation Law. In recent years they extended the services to include the care of ordinary sickness of employees. The costs of the care for workmen's compensation are, of course, borne by the employer under the legal requirements of the state. The costs of medical care for the nonservice-connected injuries or disabilities are borne jointly by the employer and by the employee through a monthly deduction from salary. The insurance companies make agreements with designated physicians and hospitals to serve policyholders according to an agreed fee schedule, the fees being paid by the insurance companies. As a rule, these policies are available only to groups of employed persons through the sponsorship of the employer.

Recently some casualty insurance companies in California and a few companies specially organized for sickness insurance have offered policies which may be sold to individuals, but which are sold at lower rates to organized groups of employees at a fixed amount per year per member. These types of policies have been ruled in California as legally constituting "service contracts," and not as contracts of insurance, subject to regulation by the state insurance department. As a result, some irresponsible fly-by-night companies have been organized, with resulting injury to the health of the people as well as to medical professions and institutions.

In some cases, as in Roanoke Rapids, North Carolina, several enterprises have combined to provide all their employees and their families with medical and hospital care, supported jointly by regular payments through deductions from wages and contributions from the employer. As a result, this type of medical service takes on the nature of a community medical service, particularly in view of the fact that the employees of the three textile mills which support the medical service comprise the bulk of the wage-earning members of this community. One of the most comprehensive industrial medical services in the United States at the present time with direct charge against the treasury of the company is that provided at the Endicott-Johnson Shoe Company, Binghamton, New York. This organization in 1928 provided free medical care for fifteen thousand employees and the dependent members of their families. There are no restrictions on the kind or amount of medical care which any individual may receive.

University Medical Services

A more recent development in group payment for medical care is the service to the students of the leading universities and colleges in the United States. Beginning with physical examinations or treatments connected with participation in athletic exercises, the services have expanded to include first aid for general illnesses and finally complete medical service, including both preventive and curative phases. Usually the students pay a fixed amount for medical services, which is included in tuition fees. The amounts of service and the annual fees vary with the particular institutions. A few institutions have recently given serious consideration to the problem of extending the benefits of the university medical services to faculty members and to their families. At the present time at the University of Minnesota such benefits are extended in a limited degree to members of the faculty. At the University of Chicago, all the staff and employees of the University Clinics receive medical care on the payment of a fixed monthly amount.

Annual Medical-Service Agreements

There are, of course, many persons not connected with factories or institutions large enough to support a complete medical service. Smaller groups, therefore, have relied upon voluntary agreements with medical practitioners and institutions for specific types of medical care to individuals requiring it in consideration of regular payments from all members of the group. Usually these groups have been employees of the same business enterprise. Several types of these voluntary agreements will be described as illustrative of the different forms of organization which may be applied. It will be noted that some of the employed groups receive subsidy from the employer, whereas others do not; some of them provide for a maximum cost to the group, regardless of the amount of service, and all provide for regular payments by the individual regardless of the medical benefits he may receive personally.

In Dallas, the Employees' Mutual Benefit Association of the street railway company has arranged for a monthly pay-roll deduction to provide money benefits and medical care by physicians during periods of sickness or disability other than those covered by the Workmen's Compensation laws. (Money benefits and medical care for compensable accidents are provided by the employer.) There are about eight hundred members of the employees' association who pay eighty-five cents per person per month for professional services by the physicians of a well-known clinic in the city of Dallas. In addition to this contribution the company makes a payment of one hundred dollars per month with the resulting average of about one dollar per month per person for professional services at the offices of the clinic or by the physician members of the clinic when patients are hospitalized. The monthly payment does not cover home calls or the costs of hospitalization. The costs of hospitalization are met in part, however, from the monthly deductions, the employees' association paying directly to the hospital a maximum sum of thirty dollars for services to members. The remainder of the hospital charge is borne by the individual himself.

Approximately 98 per cent of the employees of the street railway company are members of the association, the other 2 per cent being transient workers or those who for particular reasons are not eligible for the benefits of the mutual association. The contract has been in effect for a period of five years and is generally regarded as satisfactory by the employees and by the physicians doing the work. The average income of the employees of this association is in the general neighborhood of one hundred dollars per month. Similar annual medical-service agreements between electric railways employees' associations are in effect in Houston and Fort Worth.

A somewhat different type of agreement prevails for the employees of a well-known steamship line with headquarters at San Francisco and at Seattle. At Seattle, approximately one thousand persons are employed by the steamship line and are required individually to agree to a monthly deduction of one dollar and a half for the cost of medical care to themselves. The medical care includes complete service for the individual except for tuberculosis, nervous and mental conditions, and venereal diseases. No service is available to the family, and no house calls are made without extra charge to the individual. Hospital services are provided at no extra cost to the extent of twenty-one days in any one calendar year. The agreement is drawn between the employer and a clinic comprising fourteen physicians who conduct a private hospital of two hundred beds. Services must be rendered, except in emergencies, by these physicians and in this hospital. At the time the annual medical service was instituted, participation was voluntary on the part of the employees. It was understood, however, that all future employees would agree to participate in the group-payment plan for medical care.

Inclusive Medical Service

A more inclusive scheme involves an agreement between the employees' association of Los Angeles County and a clinic in the city of Los Angeles. In this city more than three thousand families are covered by an annual medical-service agreement at a cost of two dollars per month per wage-earner member, regardless of the size of his family. Payments are made to the clinic monthly by the secretary-treasurer of the association, at the established rate per certified member. Not all members of the association subscribe for the medical services. Association dues are collected by monthly pay-roll deductions. No contributions are made by the employer toward the costs of the medical services.

For members complete medical care is provided, including the services of doctors, nurses, hospitals, and outside consultants when necessary. Not more than three months' hospitalization will be given to any one particular individual during a twelve months' period. No types of diseases are excluded from treatment, although the group of medical practitioners agrees to treat tuberculosis cases only until they are committed to a tuberculosis sanitarium and mental cases only until they are committed to a government institution. The patient is required to pay for his own medical supplies and appliances such as insulin, eyeglasses, and crutches.

House calls are charged for at a nominal rate, sufficient to prevent abuse of the privilege by members. The cost of hospitalization for family members must be borne by the patient himself and is not included in the agreement with the clinic.

Recently the clinic has also arranged for agreements with other employees' associations in the city, particularly those employed by the city of Los Angeles, namely, the waterworks employees and the police and firemen. It is interesting to observe here that one single medical group has contracted with a number of different employees' associations.

At the city of Fort Smith, Arkansas, a somewhat different arrangement was put into effect where a special medical and protective association was organized, memberships being secured from the employees of various industries in the city and in the vicinity. The association arranges for medical care from physicians and hospitals in the community at a rate of two dollars per month per family. Each certificate-holder is entitled to complete medical care for his family including hospitalization. During the year 1931, fifty-eight hundred memberships were in effect and more than five thousand hospital days of care were given to certificate-holders and to their families. Certain restrictions are placed upon the amount of service which any one employee or family member may receive as well as on the types of benefits which are available.

Hospital Insurance

Of special interest to hospital superintendents are the various forms of hospital insurance now in effect in the United States. For at least ten years attempts have been made to institute hospital-insurance plans by which individuals may pay a fixed sum and be guaranteed hospital care in one of several institutions. One kind of plan is that by which a promoter organizes a hospital association for the sale of individual policies. In such cases the association pays the hospital used by a policyholder for all services covered by the insurance agreement. The hospital bears no financial risk and has no financial assurance, except for the payment of certain bills by the association. Plans of this type, when organized for profit, have not succeeded. Some groups, however, organized as not for profit have continued in existence for several years, notably the Rockford (Ill.) Hospital Association and the Thomas Thompson Trust of Brattleboro, Vermont. Each of these associations has been in operation for more than ten years, and has more than three hundred policyholders under contract.

A more recent and comprehensive hospital-insurance plan has been that in which the hospital contracts with a group of policyholders directly or through an association to provide certain definite services at an agreed sum per person per year. In Dallas, Texas, two hospitals, the Baylor and the Methodist, each have under contract several thousand employed persons. The terms of the contracts vary in slight detail, but for the purposes of the present discussion, the agreements may be described as follows: For the payment of fifty cents per person per month, the hospital agrees to provide, without extra charge, hospital service when needed, including operating-room service, anesthetics and laboratory fees, routine medicines, surgical dressings, and hypodermics for a period not to exceed twenty-one days during a twelve months' interval. After twenty-one days the beneficiary is given a one-third discount on regular and special hospital services required during an illness. The benefits of the plan do not include X-ray service, special prescriptions, serums, or doctors' or special nurses' fees, although liberal discounts are granted from the usual fees for X-ray services.

Contagious, tuberculosis, and mental cases are not included in the benefits, after they have been diagnosed as such. Obstetrical cases are granted 50 per cent discount on hospital services after a period of ten months' membership. In case no beds are available in the hospital, patients will be cared for in another institution. In cases of a general epidemic causing a lack of beds throughout the entire city, the hospital will refund to persons needing hospitalization twice the amount paid during the previous twelve months. Except for accidents, which are taken care of immediately, the contract becomes operative ten days after date of application.

The financial arrangements provide a minimum of expense to the hospital. Groups of employees join in subscribing to the hospitalization plan. They collect the monthly, quarterly, or semi-annual dues and make one single payment. Individuals are not permitted to join the plan singly, nor may individual members pay their fees directly to the hospital.

About forty groups, ranging from ten or fifteen members to more than two thousand members, are under contract with the Baylor Hospital for hospital service. No promotion expense is incurred by the hospital for the sale of insurance agreements, although the bookkeeping in connection with collections from groups is carried on through the offices of the hospital. The first agreement for hospital services was drawn between the Baylor Hospital and a group of teachers in the Dallas city schools. The rate for school-teachers was recently raised to eight dollars per year, although the six-dollar rate has proved satisfactory to other groups. The success with this group led to applications by other employed groups, particularly city employees. At present, employees of banks, department stores, insurance companies, newspaper publishers, wholesale houses, brokerage concerns, and others are under contract.

Summary

It may be surprising to some hospital people that a sum as small as fifty cents per month is adequate to remunerate the hospitals for the services to members. Whether this amount would be too large or too small for certain groups or communities could, of course, be tested only by experience. But several features of the group-hospitalization plan operate to make it financially advantageous to the hospital. First, a minimum revenue is assured through the regular contributions by the group, whereas many of the patients would otherwise have been accepted as charity cases. Second, the patient is required to pay for his own X-ray service and does not, therefore, request unnecessary treatment. Third, the limit of twenty-one days for care protects the hospital against large expense for chronic or incurable cases. Fourth, the additional cost of giving board-and-room service to a patient in a hospital which is ready to serve at full capacity is often very low. Fifth, the privilege of refunding money in case of an epidemic avoids the possibility of the plan's being a financial drain on the hospital.

What is the effect of a group-payment plan upon the quality of medical care received and the professional status and dignity of the physicians and hospitals providing the services? This question is an important one. If the assurance of a stated revenue, or the inadequacy of the remuneration, results in impersonal or superficial medical services by physicians or hospitals, the group-payment plan will ultimately be detrimental to the patients it is intended to benefit. Some group-payment plans appear to benefit both patients and the medical practitioners and institutions. Others appear to be unsatisfactory to all groups concerned, from the scientific as well as the financial point of view. The interests of both the professions and the public must be considered in the provision of medical care. Where the medical practitioners and institutions are adequately remunerated, where the working conditions are such as to maintain a high quality of service, where the costs to a group of members are not increased unduly by overhead costs or abuse of the privilege—where these conditions exist, the group-payment principle of sickness insurance yields advantages to both the medical profession and the public.

The foregoing illustrations all show the application of the insurance principle on a voluntary basis. There is, at present, in the United States, no legal compulsion upon groups to carry sickness insurance, except in connection with workmen's compensation agreements. To be sure, some of the plans are virtually compulsory upon the employees of firms, the compulsion being exerted either by the employer or by the members of the employees' associations.

Sickness insurance, even compulsory sickness insurance, is to be sharply differentiated from state medicine. Sickness insurance is a device by which people pay for their own medical care. It has no necessary connection with state subsidy through the collection of taxes or with medical care by government doctors or hospitals. Even in some countries in Europe the sickness-insurance organizations are independent of government subsidy or control. It is well to point out, however, that the use of tax money for the payment of medical bills is also a method of "group payment" for the costs of medical care. Insurance is a device by which a group of people pay for their own medical care. Taxation is a device by which one group pays for another group's medical care.

Sickness insurance is a plan by which self-supporting people continue to remain self-supporting as a group as well as individually. It is not a means of dispensing charity. It is a means of avoiding charity.

During the year 1932, I visited and corresponded with many of the new hospital-care insurance plans being developed throughout the nation, and there resulted the following article, which appeared in the January 1933 issue of the magazine The Modern Hospital. *Later that year, I obtained permission from my employer, the Julius Rosenwald Fund, to serve as part-time consultant to the Council of the American Hospital Association, which had formally approved the sponsorship of group hospitalization. This article discusses some fiscal, professional, social, and organizational aspects of group hospitalization, at a time when there were no authorities to be consulted or literature to be studied.*

Group Hospitalization: Mecca or Mirage?

The present widespread interest in group payment for hospital service—voluntary hospital insurance—is not accidental. It is fundamental. For several years the difficulty of the hospital in collecting patients' fees and the difficulty of the individual patient in paying for hospital service have suggested the need of stabilizing hospital revenue.

Group hospitalization plans have been instituted or are in contemplation in a number of cities, among them Dallas, Fort Worth, San Antonio, Shreveport, Louisville, New Orleans, Colorado Springs, Pueblo, Newark and Elizabeth, N. J., New York City, Philadelphia, Brattleboro, Vt., Grinnell, Iowa, and Rockford, Ill. The following discussion will be based upon the experiences and special features of the various types of group hospitalization schemes represented in these cities.

The explicit recommendations of the Committee on the Costs of Medical Care in favor of voluntary hospital insurance will undoubtedly give impetus to the study and development of such plans. From the standpoint of the hospital patient, the plan of ensuring the payment of his hospital bill through fixed monthly dues removes the uncertainty of such costs and of the ability to meet them.

It is not the purpose of this article to discuss the theoretical advantages and limitations of group hospitalization to the institution or the patients. The experiences of hospitals that have instituted the plan show that each hospital must solve its own problems with regard to such features as the monthly or annual premium, the type and scope of medical benefits, and the enlistment of support by medical practitioners. The unanimous testimony of hospital administrators who have experimented with the group payment plan appears to be about as follows: Physicians ultimately, if not immediately, recognize that group hospitalization increases the possibility of collecting a reasonable medical or surgical fee. Patients and physicians do not abuse the privilege of free hospital service merely because it is paid for in advance. The receipts for premiums exceed the fees which probably would have been collected from the same individuals for the same amount of hospital service. The increased revenue to the hospitals from group hospitalization exceeds materially the increased expense from serving such subscribers.

On the following pages I wish to consider certain practical administrative features of putting a group payment plan into operation, assuming that it is regarded as theoretically sound and socially desirable from the standpoint of a particular institution. The following points will be presented in order: (1) relative merits of individual against group policies for subscribers to the plan; (2) comparative advantages of one as opposed to several participating hospitals; (3) proprietary *versus* nonprofit promoting and administrative organization; (4) relations with medical staffs; (5) scope of hospital benefits; (6) types of illnesses covered; (7) methods of remunerating participating hospitals for services to patients; (8) legal aspects of group hospitalization.

Large Group Contracts Are Best

By group hospitalization is meant a plan by which a large number of individuals contribute equal amounts to a common fund which is to be used for purchasing hospital service for members who require it. Ordinarily hospital service applies solely to the care of bed patients (excluding outpatient care), and has no connection with fees to, or the professional services of, attending physicians or surgeons. The hospitals individually or as groups guarantee to provide medical service under the terms of the contract regardless of the amount of premiums collected; all premiums or dues paid by subscribers are paid to the hospital or hospitals, regardless of the amount of service rendered. Group hospitalization of this type is to be distinguished from arrangements by which private clinics or private insurance companies collect premiums or dues. The private clinics or commercial insurance companies either pay to the policyholders fixed daily sums, regardless of the hospital bill, or make cash payments to the hospitals for services rendered according to a basic fee schedule. Plans of the latter type are in effect in Little Rock, Los Angeles, San Diego, Portland, and Seattle, to mention a few cities.

A group hospitalization plan should center its emphasis upon group insurance agreements rather than upon contracts with separate individuals. The sale of a hospitalization contract to an individual involves high sales expense, high cost for office administration and bookkeeping, and a repetition of sales effort at the time of the renewal of each policy. When individual contracts are offered it is usually the more sickly who are most apt to recognize the benefits of the plan. Consequently the subscribers include a relatively large number of "bad risks" from the financial point of view.

Another difficulty with individual contracts is that policyholders are not previously known to or acquainted with each other. Consequently even though hospital benefits are received by a reasonable proportion of the subscribers, these facts are not known to other policyholders in the same way as if they were members of the same industrial, social, or political group. It is a good idea for Mr. Jones to know when his fellow employee, Mr. Smith, goes to the hospital as a beneficiary of the group hospitalization plan. The psychological effect of observing one's neighbor receive hospital benefits under the plan is lost when the individual subscribers are not known to each other.

When group policies rather than individual policies are written, one sales effort suffices to enroll a number of people employed by a factory or mercantile enterprise. The members of the group talk the plan over among themselves, and the individual subscribers consciously or unconsciously influence others to increase the membership. Collections for a group may be made through an employer or through the secretary of an employees' association. Renewals for the group do not require solicitation. They may be handled through the device of merely allowing subscribers to continue to pay subscriptions, in advance, for the period of time to be covered.

The most satisfactory groups for hospital insurance are obviously the large ones because of the reduced office expense for bookkeeping concerning the collection of dues. The subscribers should also be more or less homogeneous in social and economic status, so that individuals will agree in their appraisal of benefits received. The employees of a factory or members of a trade union "local" would be particularly satisfactory in this respect.

Individual Policies More Risky

It is especially desirable that relatively high proportions of each group be enrolled as subscribers. The hospitals should insist, if possible, that at least 50 per cent of any group applying for group hospitalization benefits should subscribe for and join the plan. In this way "adverse selection" of subscribers would be avoided. An unduly high proportion of "bad risks" might cause either a loss to the hospitals or an increase of premiums to the subscribers. Special discounts from the standard "dues" may be allowed for large groups, and for groups in which a high percentage of the eligible members became subscribers.

Individual policies can be made acceptable in some instances by requiring a physical examination or a waiting period before a subscriber is entitled to hospital benefits. Individual memberships should also carry larger premiums and should be payable on a semiannual or annual basis. Moreover, individuals should probably be accepted only upon application rather than being aggressively solicited. By such arrangements as these the individual subscribers can be accepted without jeopardizing the financial stability of the plan.

Should a single hospital attempt a group hospitalization plan or should it participate with other local institutions? This question cannot be answered categorically. A single hospital would of course receive more revenue from group hospitalization if it were not required to share with others in the payments on behalf of sick subscribers. On the other hand, the total number of subscribers would probably be greater if several institutions participated in the group hospitalization scheme.

Cooperative Plan Is Preferable

For one hospital to succeed with group hospitalization, it should maintain an open medical staff. Even then, unless attending physicians preferred the particular hospital sponsoring the plan, the scheme might be hindered materially through public opinion and the opposition of the medical profession.

Participation by a group of hospitals is, in general, preferable from the public as well as from the professional point of view. Such participation is necessary if the patient is to have reasonably free choice of a physician at the time of hospitalization.

There is nothing about the joint action of several hospitals that would interfere with existing professional or personal privileges in the respective institutions. Group hospitalization would not compel a hospital to allow a physician to attend a subscriber unless such a physician were a member of the attending staff or courtesy staff for the type of service required. Nor would it be required for a hospital to accept a patient unless the subscriber were eligible, under ordinary conditions, for the services and type of accommodations required.

Physicians and patients naturally would prefer some institutions to others, a preference that now exists in any community. Subscribers and physicians would use those hospitals which, in their opinion, provided the greatest benefits in exchange for premiums paid. It would be assumed, of course, that the benefits were identical in all institutions, that is to say, all institutions would provide nursing service and special services under the same conditions and with the same restrictions.

A group of hospitals could among themselves provide the working capital for a group hospitalization scheme. This burden conceivably might deter individual institutions from initiating the plan. To be sure a commercial agency might offer to finance such a plan, either at the outset or permanently.

Should the initiation and administration of a group hospitalization plan be carried on directly by the participating institutions, or should such responsibilities be delegated to a separate enterprise organized for profit? The answer lies in the comparative economies of the two methods, having in mind such factors as the availability of an efficient executive or salaried manager, the source of original working capital, and the probable expenses of bookkeeping and administration. One thing is clear: The method of promotion must be such that no individual or group of individuals can gain personally through the decrease or restriction of the medical services required by the subscribers. The payments to the participating hospitals must be a definite total sum irrespective of the total volume of service required from them. Payments to employees or middlemen must not be allowed to influence the amount and quality of medical services rendered.

Most of the contractual arrangements have been effected through agencies that receive a definite commission on the premiums collected. This stated commission avoids the danger of the promoting agency's attempting to influence payments out of the common fund to the individual participating hospitals.

The question of the desirability of using a proprietary sales and administrative agency for group hospitalization is not to be settled on mere theory. It is a practical problem for each group of hospitals to consider along the following lines: Could the group of hospitals through their own organization with employed executives protect their own professional practices in the community more satisfactorily than a commercial sales agency? Could a nonprofit association of the participating hospitals develop as large and as economically desirable a total of subscribers as the middleman?

The Administrative Costs

With regard to the first question, the scale would appear to tip in favor of the hospital's own organization. With regard to the second question, matters of local custom and available personnel would be the immediate deciding factors. The special qualities of the private promoter may make him admirably suited to introduce the group hospitalization plan to employees and groups of employers in any particular community. On the other hand, the employment of a paid executive by the hospitals themselves might involve lower overhead costs with equally satisfactory results.

It has been customary for proprietary agencies to receive for their services from 30 to 40 per cent of the premiums collected. Some agencies have arrangements by which lower percentages are received after a twelve-months' period from the enrollment of the respective individual or groups of subscribers. Usually 10 per cent is paid as a commission to the salesmen, and from 20 to 30 per cent is used for administrative costs, office upkeep, and profit. A financially sound enterprise sponsored by a group of hospitals probably could in many instances reduce the proportionate overhead costs, and in this way offer the service at lower premiums to patients or make possible higher payments to the participating hospitals. It is possible also that a nonprofit organization may receive more favorable publicity in the local press, as well as economically valuable support from influential citizens, particularly hospital trustees.

Help of Medical Staff Needed

The promotion of a group hospitalization plan must be aggressive. The public will see the theoretical advantages but will be suspicious of the practical workings. Some people still remember various fly-by-night attempts at group hospitalization which have been promoted on unsound financial bases during the past twenty years. The benefits must be explained clearly and continuously to groups of prospective subscribers. Such promotion costs money, and must be paid for directly by the hospitals and indirectly by the patients. It is for each community to decide whether it is more desirable immediately and in the long run to form a nonprofit organization to promote voluntary hospital insurance, or to turn the financial and administrative responsibilities (as well as the opportunities for gain or savings) to proprietary middlemen.

The medical staff of any particular hospital should, of course, be sympathetic to group hospitalization if the plan is to be launched under the most favorable auspices. It is important that a hospital director participating in such a scheme explain the idea and workings of group hospitalization, so that physicians may aid in establishing proper attitudes among actual and prospective subscribers.

A doctor would in most instances find it easier to collect a reasonable fee from subscribers who became his patients than from the same persons if they were required to pay hospital bills from their private resources. Moreover, the doctor is given reasonable freedom in ordering diagnostic services according to the patients' needs, knowing that certain of these services will require no extra cost.

The personal relations between physician and patient would not be affected by group hospitalization. The patient would tend to be served in the hospital preferred by his physician, and the physician would have the same privileges with regard to certain types of medical service that he enjoys in the treatment of other cases. Group hospitalization would neither help nor hinder the activities of a physician with no existing hospital appointments. It would, of course, be a disadvantage to doctors whose hospital appointments were exclusively in institutions not participating in the group payment plan, for patients would be accepted by the hospitals only when attended by physicians eligible to serve in the respective institutions.

A question arises concerning the care of patients who are unable to pay physicians' or surgeons' fees, even though the group hospitalization dues would remunerate the institution for the hospital benefits. This situation would remain the same as at present. A physician bringing his patient to the hospital would know in advance whether or not he intended to make a charge for his services. The doctor would make his choice of serving this patient personally on a no-charge basis or referring him to members of the attending staff who were "on service" for nonpaying patients.

The amount and type of hospital benefits will vary with the premium to be charged and vice versa. Group hospitalization plans have ranged in their fees from six to twelve dollars, and in their medical benefits from twenty-one days board and room and the use of the operating room only, to thirty days complete hospital care, including unlimited X-ray and laboratory services, as well as blood transfusions. The scope of the benefits and the annual premiums must be decided on the basis of estimated future expense and the psychologic effect of certain inclusions or exclusions. In general, it seems that the additional charge necessary for certain special benefits, such as X-ray, are more than offset by the sales appeal attendant upon offering an inclusion of these with very few exceptions. The benefits should in every instance include the basic necessities that most patients require, such as a certain number of days of board and room service and the use of the operating rooms.

The Matter of "Extras"

With regard to special services, such as X-ray, laboratory, basal metabolism tests, physicians may vary in their professional judgment as to the necessity of these procedures in a given case. One of three financial policies may be adopted by the participating hospitals with regard to these socalled "extras": (1) the premium may be increased sufficiently to cover the estimated total costs of special services, assuming there will be some "unnecessary" work; (2) special services may be offered to subscribers at a proportionately reduced rate, regardless of the amounts purchased; (3) special services may be charges at standard rates with an agreed maximum total fee regardless of the benefits received. Each of these three policies has been adopted with success in different institutions. The first of them would appear to be most satisfactory from the point of view of subscribers, even though it may result in a higher total monthly payment by each member of the group. In this way the costs of the more expensive illnesses would be distributed over all subscribers rather than centered upon those requiring hospitalization.

Certain Illnesses Usually Excluded

Group hospitalization is most useful and most needed in the care of acute and unpredictable illnesses of relatively short duration. These include all forms of accidents and functional disorders requiring bed care or surgery. It is common for group hospitalization plans to exclude illnesses which are chronic, predictable, or avoidable. The expenses of such illnesses are borne by taxes or are thrown back on the individual as "punitive damages." Usually chronic diseases, such as tuberculosis, mental diseases, arthritis, and cardiac troubles require bed care only in their last stages and at a time when the patient himself is not a self-supporting member of his own community. Predictable disease, more or less within the individual's control, such as alcoholism, venereal disease, willfully self-inflicted injuries and pregnancy, must be treated by office care in the early stages and require bed care only under conditions that can be foretold several months in advance.

The exclusion of tuberculosis, mental disease, and venereal diseases does not mean that such cases should not be covered through group payment, but rather that they should be made the responsibility of an entire community rather than of a particular small group in which the proportion of individuals suffering from these conditions would not be uniform. It is customary for subscribers to group hospitalization plans to receive special discounts for maternity service and for the treatment of willfully self-inflicted injuries. The hospitalization of infectious cases is usually excluded, as being more appropriate for provision in local governmental institutions.

In determining the methods of payment by individual subscribers a choice must be made between frequent payments which minimize the financial burden upon the subscriber and infrequent payments which minimize the bookkeeping for the receipt of funds by the participating hospitals. It is particularly desirable that any unpaid installments be demanded at the time a subscriber receives medical services and that he be required to pay in full for the entire fiscal period, usually a year, during which he receives any or all of his hospital benefits. The determination of the fiscal year may provide for a twelve-month period from the date of enrollment or a date from some particular day of the year for all patients, such as January 1 or July 1.

Payments to hospitals on behalf of subscribers admitted for service should insofar as possible be on a flat rate all-inclusive basis, with no extras. This should mean that a hospital would receive no more cash for a case which required a great deal of special service than for one requiring only board and room care. Consequently some cases would be relatively more profitable to the hospitals than others, but in the long run the income to the hospitals would be balanced according to the amount of service rendered.

The amount of the daily payment to the hospital will depend upon previous agreement and will be influenced by the size of the monthly premiums. The daily allowances might deliberately be set at a figure lower than that estimated to consume the entire premiums, with a provision for periodic distribution among the participating hospitals according to days of care rendered. For example, the immediate payments to hospitals might be three, four, or five dollars a day, even though the dues would have been sufficient to pay at the rate of eight dollars a day of care.

An agreement would also be necessary for a pro rata reduction in the daily payments to hospitals in case an epidemic or other calamity required the acceptance of an unusually large number of subscribers. Usually the conditions increasing hospital admissions would not apply to all subscribers at once or to subscribers only. An accident would not affect all subscribers; likewise an epidemic of influenza would not be limited to them. The increased admission of subscribers suffering from an epidemic disease would be attended by increased income from private patients and a lower per capita operating cost from increased utilization. The reduced proportionate payments to participating hospitals on behalf of subscribers would therefore not be a total loss to the institutions.

Privileges Not Generally Abused

The economic effects of a group hospitalization plan must be determined by comparing the receipts on behalf of subscribers with any of the three following amounts: the prices ordinarily charged for the services received by the individual subscribers; the per capita costs of the institution as a whole; the additional costs entailed by services to subscribers. The last-mentioned amount—the increase in the total hospital expense budget—is, of course, the basic figure against which each hospital should compare receipts on behalf of hospitalized subscribers. Most hospitals have found and probably will find that the revenue received from group hospitalization is greater than that which would have accrued to the hospital for the same services to the same patients.

It may be feared that patients and attending physicians will demand unnecessary services. This possibility, although a real one, has not proved to be serious in practice. In the long run both physicians and patients have shown a desire to limit hospital benefits to those necessary to good medical care and have not abused the privileges to which they were entitled.

Legal Advice Should Be Sought

As ordinarily set up the agreements represent "contracts" by the hospitals, individually and severally, to render certain professional "services" and not to pay or to guarantee to pay certain amounts of "money." Consequently, in several states group hospitalization has not been regarded as coming under the insurance laws, but has been regulated by the common law regarding contracts of service. The responsibility to render service rests upon the hospital which accepts the individual subscriber, and the service must be rendered by the hospital regardless of whether it is paid for by the central fund. If facilities are not available in one institution, because of crowded conditions or medical policy, the responsibility shifts to another hospital. In case all hospitals are occupied to capacity the association may discharge its responsibilities by paying a specified sum, such as a multiple of the annual premium, to each patient requiring hospitalization during the period. . . .

Skillful Management Is Required

Group hospitalization is economically sound in practice. The group payment plan provides an equitable distribution among subscribers of the costs of hospital care. The revenue from subscribers tends to stabilize and increase a hospital's income from patients of limited means. The promotion and management of a group hospitalization scheme, however, are not simple procedures and should not be embarked upon in a light-hearted manner. They require careful study and skillful management. They require an understanding of the problems of professional relations with physicians, of community relations with patients, and of the economics of hospital service. Properly planned and managed, group hospitalization may be a genuine economic benefit both to hospitals and to the public. Its development throughout the country and in particular localities will depend upon the foresight and administrative skill of hospital superintendents and trustees.

At the September 1934 American Hospital Association convention in Philadelphia, when I was an Associate for Medical Services of the Julius Rosenwald Fund, Chicago, I presented my second annual report as a part-time consultant to the Council on Administrative Practice and Community Relations of the American Hospital Association. The following paragraphs are excerpts from the report.

A Model Plan for Group Hospitalization

Group hospitalization is a way of putting hospital care in the family budget. It is not primarily a way of putting money into the hospital budget. The public has no particular interest in problems of hospital finance, but the ordinary citizen has a lively interest in the problem of his personal finance. Group hospitalization is a way by which people pay hospital bills and not a way by which the hospital pays its own bills. . . .

Group hospitalization applies the principle of insurance, of removing the uncertainty of a large hospital bill and replacing it with the certainty of a small hospital bill. . . . No one can tell when he is going to be sick or what his sickness will cost him. If he could tell, there would be no discussion of group hospitalization. . . .

The average cost of medical care is not high; the average cost of hospital care is not high. . . . But if a bill of $65 or $165 is presented to a patient, it is no comfort to the patient to know that hospitals are well managed. He is interested only in some plan by which he can pay the hospital bill. . . .

It is sometimes said that if people would be as careful about budgeting their hospital bills as they are about keeping up their installments on the radio and automobile, we would not have all this talk about the cost of hospital care. This is true. But the individual's sickness is unpredictable. On the other hand, the sickness of a group of individuals can be predicted with reasonable accuracy. . . . It is possible for a group of people to do what is impossible for an individual, namely, to place hospital care in the family budget. . . .

Group hospitalization, as officially endorsed by the American Hospital Association, applies to hospital bills only. The question of the inclusion of the physician's fee is often raised by members of the general public as well as by physicians. The question may be answered this way: "Whenever physicians want their fees included it will be done."

One-third of the population requiring hospital care for acute ill-nesses receives it at government expense or through philanthropy. In 1929 not more than five percent of the people were receiving relief for food, clothes, and shelter, yet a third of the people were receiving relief in the form of hospitalization. The standards of ability to pay for hospitalization are different from those for ability to buy economic commodities which can be budgeted. . . .

How far down in the economic scale must you go before you find a person who cannot pay a hospital bill? One-third of the population is now receiving free hospital care. Who cannot afford to subscribe to a group hospitalization plan at five, six, seven, or eight dollars a year? Only the unemployed. . . .

An acquaintance of mine who is on "relief" explains that he now rolls his own cigarettes. In this way he makes a 5-cent package last two days. Five cents every two days, two and a half cents a day, is about $9.15 a year—more than the rate for a group hospitalization plan providing semi-private accommodations. . . .

I do not say that people should give up tobacco for hospitalization. I merely say that hospital care could be budgeted (and should be budgeted) along with sweets, chewing gum, and tobacco, without the aid of governments or philanthropy. . . .

The following characteristics of a group hospitalization plan are set forth as desirable features from the points of view of public welfare and hospital support:

1. Nonprofit sponsorship and control.

2. Provision of initial working capital and reserves . . . from contributions or loans, rather than from accumulation of subscriptions.

3. Lowest possible annual subscription rates. A low annual rate is desirable even if it requires limiting the subscribers' benefits to the use of the lower-priced hospital accommodations.

4. Widest possible coverage as to types of subscribers. Plans should ultimately be developed for membership by employees and families: large groups, small groups, individuals, women, children, unemployed dependents.

5. Greatest possible coverage as to special diagnostic and treatment services.

6. Minimum of exclusions as to cases accepted for hospitalization. Exclusions should be dictated by facts as to other coverage, such as workmen's compensation, or governmental provision for

mental, tuberculosis, or communicable diseases cases. Subscription rates may well include services for maternity cases, without extra charge, or at discounts from regular rates.

7. Free choice of hospital service should be available in all hospitals of standing in the community, and to some degree in other communities.

8. Adequate payments to group-hospitalization employees, on a basis which will not jeopardize quality of service.

9. A uniform schedule for remunerating hospitals, for the same types and classes of service. This may be accomplished by an all-inclusive day rate, or a schedule for each type of service, such as board and room, operating room, laboratory, X-ray, etc. The maximum liability of the association . . . should be stated in the agreement.

10. Admission for hospital care only upon recommendation of a medical practitioner and for treatment only while under his care.

11. Definite statement as to liability of participating hospitals or the hospital service association when "specific performance" of service is impossible.

12. Compliance with existing state legislation covering hospital service associations and insurance companies.

Interest in the periodic payment plan for the purchase of hospital care continues to grow. The widespread discussion among hospital executives which began two years ago, and which resulted in the official endorsement of group hospitalization by the American Hospital Association, has now spread to the medical profession and the general public.

Hardly a meeting of medical men occurs but the subject of the principle of insurance becomes one of the topics for presentation or debate. The offices of the American Hospital Association receive inquiries almost daily for the information on the development of group hospitalization throughout the United States, and I have been called upon frequently to explain or describe many of the problems of organization.

Examples of the types of organizations before which I have appeared are local, state, and county medical societies, state hospital associations, boards of trustees of individual hospitals, organizations such as the Chicago Conference of Personnel Managers, Kiwanis International, Illinois Parent-Teachers' Association, General Federation of Women's Clubs, and many others.

All of the city-wide group hospitalization plans which were in existence a year ago have continued to expand their membership. . . . In general, the single-hospital plans in cities with more than one hospital have met with stubborn resistance in the enrollment of subscribers, even where there was no criticism of the financial stability of these hospitals or the quality of professional work. In several cities where competing hospital plans are in effect, the number of subscribers has been much smaller than might have been achieved if the institutions had worked together.

During the past year, city-wide plans have been introduced in a number of places, including St. Paul, New Orleans, Washington, D.C., and Durham, N.C. . . . An interesting development of the past year is the formation of the Elkin Mutual Aid Association in Elkin, N.C., a community of approximately 2,500 urban inhabitants and 2,500 farmers. . . . In Kingston, Ontario, a special type of plan reimburses the subscriber for the payment of hospital bills rather than make payment directly to the hospital for this service.

As a result of advice and suggestions from the offices of the American Hospital Association, the Youngstown Sheet and Tube Company has established a group hospitalization plan for its own employees, modeled to a great extent on that of the Goodyear Tire and Rubber Company.

Within the last year announcement has been made of group life insurance plans with the benefits for hospital care, issued by the Prudential Insurance Company and the Equitable Life Assurance Society of New York. The former has completed a contract with the 12,000 employees of the Firestone Tire and Rubber Company and the latter with the General Tire and Rubber Company.

There is a definite trend in all voluntary nonprofit group hospitalization plans toward the inclusion of service to dependents and the liberalization of the policy to cover more types of disease and more types of care. . . .

The question whether group hospitalization is "insurance" has been replaced by the question whether it is good for the public and for the participating institutions. Legislation has been revealed in the Ohio statutes which makes it unnecessary for nonprofit hospital service corporations to be organized under the laws of insurance companies.

During the past year, enabling legislation has been enacted in New York providing for special regulation of nonprofit hospital service corporations. In the public interest, it is necessary that group hospitalization plans receive the type of regulation which will protect the interests of both subscribers and hospitals. The regulations originally established for the control of life insurance companies are not necessarily those most appropriate for the control of nonprofit hospital service corporations.

Group hospitalization in some forms will probably continue to hold the imagination and interest of the public, and will ultimately develop under some type of auspices. Whether or not the hospital will retain control of this development and keep it on a private, nonprofit basis will depend upon courage and prompt action. There is, to be sure, some financial risk in inaugurating group hospitalization plans. But this risk is small compared to the costs daily incurred for rendering services to part-pay cases and giving free care to people who would be able to and eligible to participate in group hospitalization plans.

There is need for development in the United States of contributory schemes, based on the English principle, by which the subscription rates are intended only to cover a part of the cost, the balance to be paid through taxation or philanthropy. Such plans, which might be sold at rates from two to four dollars a year, would enable subscribers to pay from half to two-thirds of the cost of services which they are now receiving free, at the expense of philanthropists and taxpayers.

It is significant that in England at the present time (1934) the hospital contributory schemes have enrolled more beneficiaries than are entitled to the services of general practitioners under the National Health Insurance Act.

In the United States, where hospital care has been regarded as a commodity rather than as a charity, the movement toward group hospitalization cannot be regarded as complete until it reaches from 15 to 20 million wage earners. If this is not developed under the auspices of nonprofit corporations, it will ultimately be developed by private insurance companies or by a system of taxation which will rest directly upon the potential beneficiaries.

Some plans have been sponsored directly by the subscribers. The function of the hospital is merely to "take the money." The fund pays the bills, according to the agreement with the subscribers. The hospital renders the service and is paid from the fund. Such a plan, of course, makes possible free choice, because the fund pays bills in any approved hospital, and not merely in those hospitals which sign a contract. . . .

It is the moral obligation of the executives and trustees of nonprofit hospitals to investigate carefully the economic and financial significance of group hospitalization plans from the standpoint of both hospital revenue and ultimate public benefits. If people of limited means are to utilize the voluntary hospitals, they must develop some plan by which hospital care can be placed in the family budget. If this is not developed, encouraged, and experimented with by executives or representatives of hospitals, it will be developed by other bodies which may not be sympathetic to the problems of hospitals and may influence hospital policies in such a way as to interfere—for the time being, at least—with the quality of professional service.

Early in the year 1939, one of the Chicago Rotary Clubs organized a "debate" on the subject of health insurance for the American people. I, *as Director of the Commission on Hospital Service of the American Hospital Association, and Morris Fishbein, editor of the* Journal of the American Medical Association *and* Hygeia, *were both invited to participate. I supported voluntary community-sponsored health care programs, while Fishbein opposed compulsory governmental bureaucracy in the health field. I affirmed the values of protection against the financial hazards of sickness and disability; Fishbein feared damage to the doctor-patient relationship and loss of individual initiative. The following article was published in the September 1939* Rotarian, *official publication of Rotary International, Chicago.*

Health Insurance: Rorem vs. Fishbein

Voluntary Plans Point the Way (by C. Rufus Rorem)

No one can tell when he will be sick, or what his sickness will cost him. This simple fact underlies the constant agitation for socialized medicine and the recurring demand for some type of health insurance.

While, on the average, the citizen of the United States spends comparatively little for the prevention and cure of disease—about $25 annually, less than he pays for tobacco, sweets, and cosmetics—still he complains about the costs of medical care. Why? Because those costs are *uncertain, unpredictable,* and almost always *untimely.*

Any family with a steady income can budget its expenditures for food, rent, clothes, even automobiles, radios, and cosmetics, but it cannot possibly foresee, and so cannot possibly budget, its necessary expenditures for medical care and hospitalization. Certainly it could earmark $25 for such use, but it might have to spend much more, say, for an unexpected appendectomy—or might have to pay for a broken leg with the monthly savings that were to have gone for the next baby. Sickness, as the head of every household is fearfully aware, can deplete the savings of a lifetime or impoverish a family for years. It is a hazard he cannot reckon in advance.

But this very uncertainty can be and is being removed by group action in which many families each contribute to a common fund which pays the bills for their medical or hospital care. The uncertainty of a large expenditure is thus replaced by the certainty of a small one— which is merely the principle of all insurance. Those who need care

are lucky to have their sickness bills paid. Those who are not sick are lucky to be well.

Health insurance is neither new nor uncommon in the United States. Probably 10 million persons have more or less complete protection under voluntary health insurance procedures. Private insurance companies offer individual accident and health policies which reimburse the policyholder for his loss of time on the job and his expenses for medical care. Railroads, mines, and lumber camps for decades have administered plans for their own employees. Many industrial enterprises and educational institutions collect regular dues from employees or students to finance medical and hospital care. Hospital service plans, to be discussed later, are growing rapidly in all parts of the country. Private groups of doctors and cooperative groups of buyers have established voluntary health insurance plans in different parts of the United States. Many fraternal orders operate contributory health plans.

Some of the plans have been very good, some rather bad. Usually the quality of care is directly proportionate to the amounts paid for the services. Health insurance is not magic. It brings no rabbits out of the hat that were not first put there by the group. One of the greatest weaknesses in the administration of health insurance in America and Europe has been the desire to get something for nothing.

The only legally compulsory health insurance in the United States is that administered under the workmen's compensation laws of the various states, covering about 10 million workers for eight hours a day. These plans provide medical care and hospitalization for all injuries or illnesses arising from employment. Costs are met from payments by the employer to a private insurance company or a state insurance fund.

The United States government operates no plans for workers' families or plans which protect the worker 24 hours a day, although the American Federation of Labor and the Congress for Industrial Organizations have both declared themselves in favor of compulsory health insurance. The only difference between them has been the unwillingness of the latter group to agree to a deduction from the worker's pay envelope for part of the cost. The American Farm Bureau Federation has actively supported voluntary hospital or health insurance, as have many business and industrial groups which view with alarm the political control that might attend legislative compulsion and governmental subsidy.

Just a year ago last month the Federal Interdepartmental Committee on Health and Welfare presented a comprehensive national health program to the National Health Conference in Washington, D. C. Prominent among the recommendations was health insurance. But the committee rightly listed several other problems as equally important: increased preventive service through public health activities, extended health service for the indigent and unemployed, improved hospital facilities for certain areas not well supplied, and unemployment compensation for workers during periods of sickness.

The National Health Bill (Senate Bill 1620), arising from the conference, contains no direct reference to health service insurance for employed persons, and it is unlikely that any of several health insurance bills now before Congress will be reported upon favorably by the Committees to which they have been referred. Compulsory health insurance bills have been introduced annually for 20 years in the various States, and those now before the legislatures have the support of organized labor. However, I am of the opinion that none will be passed this year, although the vote in California will be close.

Meanwhile throughout the United States there is developing a limited type of health insurance for hospital bills only, under special legislation which permits nonprofit associations to contract with subscribers and hospitals under the supervision of the State departments of insurance and welfare. Since 1933 nonprofit plans for hospital-care insurance have been established in more than 60 cities and communities.

The membership in nonprofit hospital service plans had exceeded 4 million subscribers on June 1, 1939, as compared with 100,000 in July, 1935. At the present rate of growth the total membership will probably exceed 6 million persons by next January. The plans are coordinated through the Commission on Hospital Service of the American Hospital Association, which administers an approval program for plans which meet and maintain certain standards of public welfare, economic soundness, and professional qualities.

No two plans are alike in detail, but all are alike in principle. Employed people pay monthly dues of 50 to 85 cents per person, and entire families are enrolled at amounts ranging from $1.25 to $2 a month, depending on the scope and nature of the benefits. Each person is entitled, if necessary, to three or four weeks of hospital service each year, usually in semiprivate rooms, including meals, nursing, operating room, laboratory, and other special services. Benefits do not cover fees to private physicians or nurses. The payment of such bills must be arranged for by the patient individually.

Each nonprofit plan is formed as a special association, with trustees selected from the hospitals, medical profession, and general public, who serve without pay as do the trustees of a university, hospital, or social agency. Subscribers are enrolled in groups through their places of employment, and employers cooperate in the collection and payment of monthly dues. Representatives of the plans are paid on a salary basis.

At the time of sickness a subscriber has free choice of any member hospital where his attending physician enjoys staff privileges. The hospital is paid an agreed amount for each day of care to the subscribers. There is no interference in the relationships among hospitals, medical staffs, and patients. An attempt is made to enlist every hospital of standing as a member institution.

The essential economic feature of the plans is the joint guarantee of service by the group of member hospitals. These institutions agree to provide the service even though the resources of the plan might be temporarily insufficient to pay the established daily rates. More than 300,000 hospital bills have been paid, and no nonprofit free-choice hospital service plan has failed to meet its obligations to subscribers.

Nonprofit hospital service plans are, as has been noted, a form of insurance, guaranteed by the participating hospitals of each community, which in turn are supported by the general public. They are a substitute for government-controlled hospitalization, rather than competitors of stock or mutual insurance companies. The public now owns the hospitals of America through an investment of 3 billion dollars by way of philanthropy and taxation. The voluntary hospital service plans are an attempt to organize the public buying power on a voluntary basis, without the disadvantages of political control.

Health insurance is not the same as State medicine. State medicine in the United States is a plan by which one group—the taxpayers—finances medical care for another group—the unemployed and the indigent. Health insurance is a plan by which an employed group of people finances medical care for itself.

Health insurance is not a panacea for all matters of public health. It does not guarantee a minimum income for doctors or hospitals. It does not lower the total costs of medical or hospital care, because the beneficiaries usually demand and receive more services than formerly. It does not guarantee accurate diagnosis or adequate treatment, even from the world's best-trained medical profession and best-equipped hospitals. It does not lower the death rate or birth rate. It does not provide medical care for the indigent or unemployed. It does not raise the general wage level or equalize the uneven distribution of wealth.

What does health insurance do? It removes the hazard of sickness costs for persons covered by the plan. It provides payments to practitioners and hospitals for many services that would have been rendered without remuneration. It permits employed people to place health service in their budgets along with other necessities. It reduces the need for paternalism and charity from the doctor, philanthropist, and tax-payer. It encourages early consultation with qualified practitioners rather than the use of patent medicines and quacks. It permits doctors to treat cases without regard to immediate income from the patient. It permits orderly evolution in methods of paying sickness bills without revolutionary changes in the entire economic order. It develops a sense of individual initiative. No one wants complete security in every respect; but everyone desires to remove the causes of needless insecurity.

Most European countries have some degree of health insurance, with legally required participation by certain employed groups. In no European country have health insurance plans ever been curtailed or discontinued, although they have all been revised and many expanded. It is sometimes said that health insurance has failed in Europe. It would be more accurate to say that Europe has failed in some phases of health insurance. There plans were established against the firm opposition rather than under the guidance of medical practitioners. Consequently, many mistakes were made that might have been avoided if the medical profession had cooperated on policies and procedures.

One of the primary objectives of European plans was to restore the worker's income rather than his health. This emphasis resulted partly from the fact that State medicine was already well developed for hos-pitalized illness before the health insurance plans emerged. Consequently, the health service benefits were rather limited. For example, in England, health insurance services include only general practition-ers' service for the employee and not his family. The European plans were established to relieve the taxpayers as a group. The American objective has been to relieve the individual patient requiring care.

What are the prospects that voluntary hospital service plans will expand to include the services of practitioners in the hospitals and the homes? They are very slight. The hospitals of America are not in a position to guarantee the services of private physicians, surgeons, dentists, or nurses. Any such arrangement with the public would require the leadership and financial responsibility of the medical profession, and would need to be parallel rather than subordinate to hospital service plans. However, such an arrangement is working in Seattle, Washington. There the King County Medical Service Bureau has a panel of 300 doctors and about 40,000 employed persons enrolled in a voluntary health insurance plan. Newspaper reports indicate that several local and State medical societies are planning community-wide free-choice insurance plans for medical care open to the general public.

Voluntary groups interested in the principle of insurance, but op-posed to compulsory action by statute, have an opportunity and a chal-

94 A Quest for Certainty

lenge to develop an American plan of health insurance. Whether this will be a substitute, forerunner, or partner of a compulsory plans, time will tell.

One cannot be *for* or *against* health insurance any more than *for* or *against* the multiplication table, railroads, or philanthropy. It is neither mecca nor mirage. It is the line of march, not the goal; the means, not the end. Health insurance is a method of financing health service in a manner which will reduce the hazard of sickness costs to the individual patient or his family. If it serves this purpose in whole or in part, it is worth while. But there will always be administrative and human problems to be solved in the march toward individual security.

Maintain the Personal Doctor-Patient Relation (by Morris Fishbein)

"He who would surrender liberty for security," said George Washington in one of his important writings, "is likely to lose both." That warning is just as sound today as it was at the time of the Revolution. Then security meant the right of the individual to be free from unlawful search and seizure in his own home. Now, as we hear it discussed on every hand, it seems to mean the guaranty of food, fuel, clothing, and shelter, and freedom from the hazards of old age, unemployment, and illness.

Already the citizens of the Unites States are insured under a compulsory system against the hazards of old age and unemployment. Some would now extend that system to protect them against the hazards of sickness.

Now the chief opposition to compulsory sickness insurance rests squarely on the ground that it is compulsory, and thus represents another insidious step toward the breakdown of democracy. Consider existing conditions. In the event that a citizen finds himself unable to procure the necessities of life because of old age or unemployment, the Government returns to him the cash he has paid so that he may purchase these necessities. Bear in mind that it is always his own cash that is returned to him; social security does not create wealth—it merely redistributes money that workers earn.

The majority of the expense in such a system is paid by low-income workers. It is from their wages that the first deduction is made. The money paid by the employer in the form of tax is added by him to the price of the goods which are, in the vast majority of instances, purchased by the workers. Finally, only the workers pay income tax. The deduction from wages, already too small, of these costs tends to inhibit the ability of the worker to supply himself with the necessities of life, and thus may create more sickness than medical care can prevent or cure.

The opposition to compulsory health insurance rests also on the fact that it is not health insurance, but sickness insurance. The tendency of such plans is to provide little or nothing for preventive medicine. They attempt only to take care of those already sick. Immunization against disease is not provided by sickness insurance in any country. In no country in the world is periodic physical examination included as a part of the compulsory insurance system. Obviously, in no country could a really complete periodic physical examination be included, because the costs would be far beyond the reach of any such system.

In this connection it is important to realize that the death rates for such diseases as tuberculosis and diphtheria have declined more rapidly in this country than in those with compulsory sickness insurance systems. It should be pointed out that in the United States during 1938 the sickness and death rates were as low as or lower than those of any other great country in the world.

American medicine opposes compulsory sickness insurance because it tends to break down that initiative and ambition which are the marks of a young country going ahead, and which disappear completely when civilization becomes too old and begins to decay. The young physician in the United States who has had a medical education involving four years of medical school and one or two years of internship, looks forward to beginning a career in which his progress will depend on his ability in taking care of the sick and the extent to which he is willing to give of his utmost for his patients. In contrast, the young physician in many another country steps into a salaried job or position at a fixed income, depending on the number of people assigned to him by the State, and then begins a mechanized routine type of service that is harmful not only to his patients, but also to his own character and advancement.

Compulsory sickness insurance encourages excessive attention to minor illnesses and complaints, and thus brings about deficiencies in the care of more serious conditions. The tendency of medical care under every compulsory sickness insurance system is to encourage a mechanical, unprofessional type of service, giving a low grade of medical service to more people, but at the same time lowering the standards of medical service for all the people.

In the United States the hospital system has developed beyond anything available in any other country. We have more than 6,200 acceptable hospitals, and the vast majority of medical care is given in those hospitals which are known as nonprofit, voluntary hospitals. These have been built out of that fundamental motive in every great religion which makes the care of the sick a high moral objective. The setting up of State compulsory sickness insurance systems would inevitably tend to throw the burden of serious illness on these hospitals. As in Great Britain, they would soon find themselves bankrupted by the State system. Moreover, the building of hospitals by the Federal Government and the equipment and maintenance of such hospitals, which would make even more difficult the work of the voluntary hospitals, would tend to destroy the voluntary system.

Compulsory sickness insurance exalts administration above the problems of the doctor and patient. The German system has for years employed more administrators than physicians. The reported costs of administration in different countries vary from 10 to 20 percent of the total income of the system. The bills for administration multiply while hospitals and laboratories deteriorate. The setting up of a State system introduces incompetent political control. Finally these systems throw such a burden of forms, blanks, and red tape on the doctor that he must spend anywhere from one to two hours of each day in satisfying the desires of the administrators for records.

Under the system of insurance against old age and unemployment, the worker receives cash to provide himself with what he needs. Under all systems, however, it is proposed to handle the problem of medical care not with cash, but with service. This question of payment in cash or in service is fundamental. Social-service workers oppose payment in cash because of the fear that either the worker will exploit the Government or the physician will exploit the Government. Somehow little has been said of the possibility that social-service workers may exploit the Government. Payment in service makes impossible any accurate, actuarial calculations as to the costs of the service.

Medical costs vary. With rapid progress the costs constantly increase. Under such circumstances the quality of the service is lowered to the patient, the medical profession and the hospital exploited, or modern methods neglected. If these conditions do not supervene, the system becomes bankrupt. There are excellent examples now available of this succession of events.

The 1938–39 epidemic of influenza brought disaster to voluntary sickness insurance plans in existence in various parts of the United States, and threatens the financial status of hospitalization plans. Yet the epidemic of this year did not even approximate the scope or intensity of the influenza epidemic of 1918 or not a single insurance plan in existence in the country could have survived. Even the Government plan could hardly have survived under such circumstances.

Apparently it did not occur to the administrators to pass the increased cost along to the patients. The attempt is always made to balance the budget at the expense of either the hospitals or the doctors. The hospitals must get even by depreciating the quality or the amount of service rendered.

In the United States today, under our present system, we have reached a high degree of scientific advancement and a quality of medical service that is supreme. The chief difficulties are the inequalities in the availability of medical service of this high standard for great groups in the population. Nevertheless, the medical profession has not remained static in meeting this responsibility. Thousands of experiments are now being conducted in various parts of the country with the aid of the medical profession, leading to new methods of distribution and payment for medical service. These plans include 75 insurance hospitalization plans, 54 hospital insurance plans, 500 medical and hospital benefit organizations, 20 flat-rate hospital plans, 2,000 industrial medical-care plans, 24 sick-benefit union funds, 300 group medical-practice plans, 300 college health service plans, and 28 States in which the Farm Security Board has set up a system.

Much is heard of the three or four group plans which have been opposed by the medical profession. These plans are opposed, not primarily because they represent experiments with new forms of distribution of medical service, but because their operation has brought into the picture of medical practice business methods and commercialization which are fatal to medical science. Solicitation of patients, underbidding to secure contracts, and breaking down of the relationship between doctor and patient are three of the most serious aspects of such service. Opposition to all new plans is based wholly on the extent to which they deteriorate medical service, inhibit medical advancement, and break down confidence in the medical profession.

Every discussion of change in the nature of medical practice in the United States runs afoul of the habit of demanding an all-or-nothing policy in relationship to many human affairs. No scientific physician, and no established policy of the American Medical Association, has opposed social control where it represents the ideal method of dealing with medical problems. Already in New York some 35 percent of medical practice is State medicine or socialized medicine, most of it established with the encouragement of the medical profession. The work of the health departments in preventive medicine as applied to mankind in the mass, the sanitariums for the tuberculous, the institutions for the insane, and the clinics for the care of the indigent and those able to pay only a small part of the costs of medical service are examples of socialized medicine.

But these are far different from a system wherein every individual would be taxed under a State or Federal law for the setting up of a bureaucracy to administer complete medical service to every person in the State, or to the majority of the people who would be included under a less than $3,000 annual-income level or to one-half the people who might be included under a less-than-$2,000 income level. The forms of socialized medicine which take increasingly from the individual more and more of the responsibility for his own existence and which enter increasingly into the intimate affairs of human life must be opposed by all who treasure the life, liberty, and pursuit of happiness which mark the American democracy.

During the year 1946, a national health service program (Senate Bill 1606) was presented to the Congress and referred to the Senate Committee on Education and Labor. The following statement was presented to inform the Committee of the achievements of Blue Cross and of its potential as a participant in a national health care program. The Blue Cross Commission offered four recommendations, all of which have since become part of federal policy on health matters: federal support of health care for public assistance beneficiaries; federal grants-in-aid for special voluntary health programs; payroll deductions for federal employee participation in Blue Cross and other voluntary health insurance programs; and federal grants-in-aid for hospital construction.

The Blue Cross Story: U.S. Senate Hearings

Your chairman stated at the opening of these hearings that they were "a challenge to all who participate, a challenge that can be successfully met only by a sincere determination to try to understand the other man's point of view and to examine the problems in the light of facts rather than slogans or prejudices."

We are here to present the facts about the 21,400,000 members of Blue Cross Plans for hospital care, a program which has enrolled more participants in less time than any voluntary movement in the history of the world. We are directly concerned with the administration of voluntary health service, and its management and achievements. We are anxious to expand its virtues and remove its defects, and thus increase its service to our nation. We believe it should not disappear from the American scene as a noble experiment.

We participated 17 years ago in establishing many of the estimates which have been submitted as evidence that no one can tell when he will be sick or what his sickness will cost him. It is now generally recognized that the costs of severe illness weigh heavily upon a small number of people, whereas the larger proportion are faced with only small annual expenditures for necessary health services. The burden of sickness costs can be most effectively carried by application of the law of averages to the payment of hospital bills. The basic question before your committee is the method and degree of such application at the present time.

What Is Blue Cross?

A Blue Cross Plan for hospital service is a nonprofit corporation, a community organization, which accepts regular and equal payments from groups of members, the combined funds being used to pay hospital bills for those members requiring care. The hospital protection may be supplemented by a medically sponsored plan for medical and surgical care. The cost for hospital plan membership is approximately seventy-five cents a month per person or two dollars per family. Subscription rates for doctors' services in hospitalized cases are about the same.

The governing body of a Blue Cross Plan is a board of directors (which includes leaders from industry, medicine, labor, welfare, hospitals, agriculture, government) who serve without pay, just as do the trustees of a church, social agency, or educational institution. These persons have no financial interest in the success of the Blue Cross Plans, yet they devote many hours to professional and administrative policies. Their only reward is participation in a program of community service.

Benefits are available as hospital service rather than cash allowances. The services to subscribers are guaranteed by contracts with more than 3,500 community hospitals throughout the United States. Benefits are usually provided in semi-private accommodations, and include the special services necessary to diagnosis and treatment. Benefits are available for each family member, usually for three or four weeks of "full coverage," with extended periods at discounts from regular hospital charges.

Blue Cross Plans are supervised through an approval program conducted by the trustees of the American Hospital Association, and in the various states are regulated and supervised by the insurance department or other appropriate body. Usually the Plans have been established through special enabling acts. The American Hospital Association's requirements for approval include nonprofit organization, free choice of hospital and physician, hospital guarantee of service benefits, and representation of subscriber interests in control. The standards also provide for the establishment and maintenance of contingency financial reserves to protect the interests of subscribers and member hospitals.

It is not accidental that protection for hospital bills has expanded so rapidly throughout the nation. The hospitals of America belong to the people, and hospital service is generally recognized as a community responsibility. The $4,000,000,000 of capital investment in American hospitals has been obtained primarily through funds donated by the general public either as philanthropy or taxation. The hospitals have assumed a moral, and sometimes legal, obligation to accept emergency cases regardless of their ability to pay. Instances where a patient is refused emergency care are so unusual as to make headlines, or be the subject of editorial comment.

A hospital bill is a special hazard for the individual. It is unpredictable as to time and amount, frequently requires absence from gainful employment, and involves additional expenditures for professional care. It involves a severe physical shock, a high emotional crisis, and a large economic expenditure. No wonder we find people "speaking of their operations."

Blue Cross Enrollment Growth Rapid

Enrollment in Blue Cross has accelerated during the past few years, and particularly the last few months. Growth during the war years was not entirely due to increased employment and high wages. The three-month period ending March 31, 1946 witnessed the largest total net increase in the history of the movement; nearly 1,400,000 persons joined during that period. This growth occurred in spite of conversion from war to peacetime industry, and in spite of many strikes in certain industries where Blue Cross protection had been especially well accepted.

The percentage of population enrolled under Blue Cross has been highest in the eastern and northern states where large portions of the population are engaged in industry. Yet, of the 12 states which show a total of more than 20% of their population now protected under Blue Cross, four may definitely be said to be rural in character. In states with the highest percentage of enrollment, our statistics indicate that the proportion of enrollment in the small towns equals that of the industrial centers of the various commonwealths.

The complete cost of medical care for hospitalized illness (including physicians' services) represents approximately 50% of the average family budget for health services. Only one-tenth of the people are hospitalized in the course of a year. Yet 10% of the individuals bear 50% of the load for the costs of medical care to the employed population and their dependents.

Which is the more important—to cover the 50% of the sickness costs which represent the small bills paid by 90% of the population, or to cover the 50% of the costs loaded upon the 10% who suffer a serious illness requiring hospitalization? There is no clear-cut answer in principle, but administrative considerations are important.

Access to the facilities and personnel of a good hospital is itself a form of prevention. It removes the economic barrier, and encourages the subscriber to seek early treatment and attention.

It is desirable that patients have early and easy contact with general practitioners and specialists. Yet it has proved very. difficult to initiate and administer such benefits unless both subscribers and practitioners are thoroughly familiar with their rights and responsibilities. The problems of administering the benefits for a minior illness are more complex than for a catastrophic illness. Legislation alone will not remove the practical administrative difficulties, nor will it provide the facilities essential to a comprehensive prepayment program of health service.

Recent Developments in Blue Cross

We now turn to a set of affirmative statements which are presented to explain the progress and prospects of voluntary health programs. Frankly, we are doing much better than many of us had ever expected. Eight years ago, we were congratulated for having reached 1,000,000 subscribers. Now we are criticized for merely exceeding 21,000,000 participants. Friends and critics alike are emphasizing the unfinished task rather than the work already done.

Most of the American population is now eligible for participation in a nonprofit prepayment plan for hospital care. Nonprofit Blue Cross Plans now serve 43 states and the District of Columbia, and it is expected that the number will reach 47 by the end of the year. Residents of small towns are being protected through community enrollment; farm groups are being served through the activities of the farm bureaus, granges, and unions, and the establishment of specially organized county health improvement associations. Rural producers and consumers co-operatives also have served as enrollment and collection agencies. In many urban areas enrollment privileges for self-employed persons are being introduced, and Blue Cross is giving increased attention to those groups.

Over half of the 80 U.S. Blue Cross Plans offer complete protection for catastrophic illness through co-ordination with Plans for medical or surgical protection. This coverage does not meet the full need of the American people, but it removes most of the economic burden of sickness from the shoulders of the individual. Home and office calls also are being offered in some Plans, but the administrative complexities of these services have delayed their general inclusion in prepayment programs.

The Blue Cross program has proved adequate for the migrant population of recent years. Blue Cross Plans permit convenient transfers of memberships from one Blue Cross Plan to another, and they allow continuance of membership when a subscriber leaves his place of original enrollment. Liberal out-of-town benefits are provided. These privileges have been achieved through formal agreements among the various Blue Cross Plans.

Blue Cross Plans are representative of the entire community: employers, employees, agriculture, hospitals, the medical profession, welfare groups, and others. The social significance of this voluntary sponsorship and guidance cannot be overemphasized. It is consistent with human values derived from permitting individuals to act voluntarily in removing the uncertainty of their sickness costs. The economic and social foundation of a community hospital is as broad as the population itself. And the combined resources and support of a group of hospitals in a community or a state may be said to represent the combined resources and support of the entire public.

Hospital administrators and trustees regard themselves as administrators and trustees of public funds. The primary purpose of both Blue Cross Plans and hospitals is to maximize service for the people who have built the hospitals, who use them, and who support them. Critics of Blue Cross Plans have sometimes described them as "producer co-operatives," implying that their trustees were concerned only with maintaining the status quo of hospital operation and finance. The analogy is something less than complete. For, although the hospitals sponsor and guarantee the Blue Cross Plans which enroll potential patients, the net savings are distributable only to the subscribers as increased benefits or reduced subscription rates.

The proof of the pudding is not in the recipe. Blue Cross trustees have typically been able to strike a balance between the interests of subscribers who provide the money and the hospitals which provide the service. They have used the subscribers' funds economically, having regard for the necessity of maintaining professional standards through adequate payments.

Subscription rates are within the ability of most of the employed population to pay, as evidenced by the high participation among enrolled groups. In the metropolitan areas of the Atlantic seaboard, large numbers of the population have joined Blue Cross including many of those legally eligible for free medical and hospital care at the expense of the taxpayers. A voluntary (or compulsory) program will be least popular with a group of workers and their dependents who have been accustomed to receiving the same benefits at some other group's expense. Conversely, there is social justification for asking all regularly employed persons to make some contribution toward the costs of their own care. Employers' contributions have made possible very low costs for voluntary plans, and have brought them within the ability to pay of low-income persons.

Problems of adverse selection are being brought under control. In the early days of Blue Cross, groups were allowed to participate even though low percentages were enrolled. The values of protection are now so definitely established that higher percentages are readily obtained, as well as arrangements for payroll deduction which are so necessary for maintenance of membership. For individual enrollment of self-em-

ployed persons, other methods have been used to achieve proper enrollment and collection as well as the control of adverse selection. A
voluntary health plan must, of course, make sure that its revenue equals
its expenses. This has been a factor in developing administrative economy and restricting benefits to those which can be provided without
net losses.

There is co-ordination in service to the enrollment areas of Blue Cross. As
a general principle, only one Blue Cross Plan is established in each
enrollment area. Co-ordination in the interests of subscribers (in enrollment, payments, and benefits) has been accomplished by the management and trustees of the respective Plans.

*The scope and content of a voluntary Plan are necessarily affected by the
economic level and available facilities of the community in which the subscribers
are enrolled.* More comprehensive benefits are available in communities
with high income levels, especially industrial centers where there are
sufficient hospital beds and diagnostic equipment. These variations
permit the establishment of higher standards (which may serve as
examples) in areas where the social consciousness of the population has
been most fully developed. This variation suggests the ultimate possibility of equalization in service through the use of local, state, or national government funds. But the differences of income levels and
living standards have many causes, and will not be offset by merely
introducing a prepayment health program.

*Subscribers are responding in higher percentages and there are progressively
fewer cancellations among beneficiaries.* This results from the general tendency to grant payroll deductions among employed groups, the increasing practice of employer contributions towards costs, and the ease
of transfer and continuance of membership for enrolled subscribers.

*Wage agreements between labor unions and management are often written
to provide partial or full payment of prepaid health benefits by the employer.*
Blue Cross has been specially popular in such agreements because of
their nonprofit service-benefit features, and the policy of permitting
continuance of membership when employment is interrupted by strike,
lay-off, or change to another firm. The advantage of protection has
been demonstrated by a number of organizations during recent strikes.
Some of the larger corporations in the country have permitted employees to authorize advances during a strike or temporary lay-off. Conversely, Blue Cross Plans have often permitted protection to continue,
with the idea that payments would be made for a number of months
upon return to work.

*The largest employer in the United States (the federal government) does not
yet permit the privilege of voluntary payroll deduction.* The Blue Cross Com-

mission office receives letters daily from units of the United States government asking for the privilege of protection. Yet there are only 300,000 federal employees and their dependents participating in voluntary Plans because of the difficulties involved in handling organization and payment details through voluntary group leaders who are employees of the federal government. Mutually satisfactory arrangements are not possible without the privileges of payroll deduction. Undoubtedly the existing makeshift enrollment and collection procedures have in many instances proved to be inefficient for the government departments involved as well as for the Plans.

Overhead costs have been remarkably low, considering the rapid rate of growth. The average operating expense for the entire country, for all Blue Cross Plans, was approximately 12% of the total income during the year 1945. In some of the larger organizations with established memberships, the operating expenses are less than 10% of the total subscribers' payments. On the average, about three cents of the subscriber's dollar has been used for consumer education and enrollment activities. About nine cents has been required for accounting and billing procedures and the payment of benefits. The expenses for general administration are being reduced. Plans are now using streamlined methods for maintenance of enrollment records, authorization of hospital admissions, and other administrative economies consistent with good business practice and efficient public service.

Active sponsorship and encouragement of Blue Cross by federal, state, and local governments can reduce costs to subscribers and increase the membership throughout the country. Certain Department of Agriculture experiments were mentioned in these hearings and were described as disappointing. It was stated that, among a group of low-income farmers, only 40 to 50% of the eligible families took advantage of the privilege of voluntary prepayment for medical and hospital benefits, even though the federal government participated in the cost of the program. Initial participation in a voluntary plan by 50% of a group of low-income farmers is encouraging. Farmers are the most individualistic and independent-minded part of our entire population. Many have solved their problem of health service by going without the necessary care. If such an experiment were conducted in an urban community, among a group of low-income workers in an industrial plant, probably 85 to 95% of the employees would have enrolled. The voluntary plans are making great strides in reaching the rural population, and we hope that national agencies will continue to encourage groups in such participation.

Many of the Blue Cross Plans have increased their benefits during their period of operation without corresponding increase in subscription rates to the beneficiary. The increased benefits have been made possible through better "selection" among subscribers and decision to apply reserves to provision of immediate benefits. Blue Cross Plans are, of course, concerned with providing protection for all costs of hospitalized illness. In some cases, increased costs for labor and supplies in hospitals have necessitated increased rates to the subscribers. Usually, however, this has also been accompanied by increased benefits. But the problem of inflation and its effects upon increased cost of hospital care still faces Blue Cross and any program of health service, voluntary or governmental, if the quality and availability of care is to be increased and assured.

Voluntary plans have been accepted by many veterans as a genuine opportunity for family protection. Even though veterans are entitled to care under existing G. I. legislation, they recognize that at least three-fourths of the care in their families is received by wife and children. Moreover, Blue Cross benefits permit free choice of hospital and doctor, which are not available at the present time for nonservice-connected disabilities. Blue Cross Plans have exempted returning veterans from the group requirements imposed upon members of the general public, and thousands are being added daily to the Blue Cross rolls.

Blue Cross Plans have been recognized by government agencies as administrative units for the provision of benefits. Many Blue Cross Plans have signed formal agreements to serve as clearing-houses for medical and hospital care by private physicians and hospitals for service-connected conditions, when such care is authorized by the Veterans Administration. Suggestions have also been made that Blue Cross represent the state or local government welfare departments in providing health benefits to public assistance beneficiaries. No definite arrangements for this type of service have yet been completed, but they are under discussion in a number of states. These various procedures are, of course, merely incidental services of an agency established primarily to offer protection to regularly employed persons.

Contrasts with European Experience

It has sometimes been argued that voluntary health insurance is merely the road (or obstacle) to a compulsory plan, as in Europe. It is suggested that Americans should hurdle these obstacles (voluntary plans), and require the entire population to participate immediately in a complete program.

There are a number of differences between the American situation and the European scene. The typical voluntary health insurance plan in the European countries, before the passage of compulsory laws (no-

tably England), was a small organization with a few thousand beneficiaries. Many were essentially the ventures of private promoters,
although legally established as "mutual" friendly societies.

The United States has more participants in voluntary plans than the
combined population of Sweden, Norway, Denmark, Belgium, and
Holland, all of which have been cited as evidence of need for a nationwide plan in this country. Yet the number of American Plans is small.
And the most successful Plans—the Blue Cross—are organized on a
nonprofit basis. Each one serves a large community or an entire state.
They are co-ordinated on a national basis.

The provision of service for hospitalized illness in England and con-
tinental Europe has long been primarily a public responsibility. The
introduction of health insurance in the European countries was essentially *a method of relieving the taxpayer, not the worker.* The United States
is the only country in the world where the average man has ever assumed that a hospital bill was something for which he should be personally responsible.

Blue Cross National Program

The matter of when or whether our population is to be included in
a national program of financing health service must be decided by our
representatives, the Congress. The decision should be influenced by
matters of public necessity and convenience. We hope that the Congress
will take into account all of the factors in American life, including the
results and prospects of existing professionally and community-sponsored programs. We believe, as the chairman has so aptly stated, that
all programs should be considered in the light of facts, rather than
slogans or prejudices. It has been the purpose of this testimony to
bring some of these facts before you.

The Blue Cross Commission favors the following approach to a
health program for the American people:

1. *Complete medical care and hospitalization supported by taxation for all
    public assistance beneficiaries or indigent members of the population.* The
    provision of health service as a "right" to those already receiving
    public assistance would clarify the position of charitable organi-
    zations in the health field, particularly community hospitals. Ac-
    ceptance by government of responsibility for care of the officially
    declared indigent would permit voluntary plans to remove this
    burden from member hospitals, and hence from subscribers.

2. *Government aid in the construction of hospitals and clinic facilities in
    the areas which require such an assistance because of generally low in-
    come, sparse population, or sudden shift in the size or composition of the*

public (this feature has been recommended by the President, and is included in Senate Bill 191). Adequate facilities are a requirement of adequate care. Voluntary plans would increase in usefulness with the better distribution of hospitals and other health facilities.

3. *Grants-in-aid to state-approved voluntary health programs which are also supported by regular contributions from the beneficiaries.* Payments might be made to practitioners or institutions, or to prepayment plans under nonprofit auspices. Such government assistance would encourage enrollment, and have much the same result as legislative compulsion, but with freedom for localities to determine the timing and character of their health programs.

4. *Permissive payroll deduction for federal employees for participation in voluntary prepaid health service programs.* It might appear that this is a small portion of our population, and not a significant factor in developing a program for the country. Yet this large group of people should be entitled to the same conveniences in obtaining prepaid health service benefits as the rest of the workers in the nation. Moreover, the prestige of the national government, in recognizing the individual's right to participate on the voluntary basis, would be a strong and encouraging example to those private employers, as well as to the states and local governments, which have not yet seen fit to provide permissive payroll deductions for their own employees.

The purpose of this testimony has been to tell you enough about the character of the Blue Cross movement to explain its reputation with the American people at the present time. The Blue Cross Plans were started and have been maintained to serve a positive need. We wish their contribution to be considered on its merits. No Plan is perfect in every respect, and none is achieving every ideal of public service which its leaders recognize as desirable. We know that there is much to be done. And we also know that *administration is difficult; agitation is easy.*

It is a high tribute to voluntary plans that Blue Cross and other ventures have been mentioned so frequently in this testimony. The Senate committee and the United States Congress are to be highly commended for their sustained interest in developing a national health program for the entire population. We offer you our resources and experience, and trust that your committee will take all significant facts into consideration in making final recommendations to the United States Congress.

After 30 years of study and political activity, the British Parliament passed the National Health Act in 1946; the Act included a nationwide program of health care insurance for the entire population, to become effective July 4, 1948. On that day the national government took over the ownership and control of health care in hospitals. All physicians became employees of the National Ministry of Health. This discussion of the National Health Service was published in the November 2, 1947 issue of Philadelphia Medicine, *the official journal of the Philadelphia County Medical Society. At that time I was executive director of the Hospital Council of Philadelphia.*

Health Service in England
(It Could Happen Here)

Voluntary hospitals and private medical practice become history in England and Wales on July 4, 1948. The next morning all voluntary and municipal hospitals, with their endowments, plants, movable property, and liabilities, will be vested in the National Minister of Health, who becomes responsible for "comprehensive health service" for the entire population.

Hospitals and Health Centers

Hospitals and health centers will be staffed by salaried physicians; their salaries and other expenses of the institutions will be paid by the Minister of Health, in accord with policies and regulations developed by Regional Boards and approved by the Minister. Citizens of England and Wales may receive complete prevention and treatment services at hospitals and health centers at no immediate cost to themselves. If they wish care in private offices, they may obtain it at their own expense; likewise they may pay "extra" for private or semi-private accommodations during periods of bed-care in hospitals.

The new service is part of the National Health Act of 1946, which will be introduced simultaneously with the National Insurance Act of 1946, which provides unemployment and retirement benefits. Toward the combined program, each employed man and woman over twenty-one years of age will contribute (while employed) 4 shillings and 8 pence weekly through purchase of government stamps, about $60.00 per year. These contributions will provide about 40,000,000 pounds annually toward the combined program, of which the Hospital and

Specialist services alone will cost 155,000,000 pounds. The balance of the program will be supported through local taxes (rates) and by income taxes paid to the national treasury (exchequer).

Duties of Regional Hospital Boards

The Minister of Health will appoint 14 Regional Hospital Boards, who will establish budgets, make staff appointments, allocate income from central endowment funds, plan capital expansion, and generally co-ordinate the hospitals (other than teaching institutions) in their respective regions. Each board will be incorporated, and will comprise approximately 20 persons appointed from candidates presented by the Universities, General Practitioners, Local Authorities, and General Public.

There will be a "house committee" for each hospital, and a "management committee" for each group of hospitals with less than 1,000 beds. Expenditure budgets for each hospital will be transmitted through the Regional Board to the Minister, who will authorize payments from the exchequer for the institutions. Uniform accounting and joint purchasing will be developed.

At the national level, the Minister has an advisory Central Health Services Council, with various sub-committees on professional and technical problems. Its membership of 41 persons will include 21 physicans, and others selected from hospital administration, local government officials, dentists, mental health administrators, registered nurses, midwives, and pharmacists.

The administration of Health Services will have two main subdivisions: (a) Public health activities and general practitioner services outside of hospitals, which will be administered by local government authorities and will be furnished in or through Health Centers; (b) Hospital and Specialist services, which will include all care in hospitals by general practitioners, consultants, or specialists.

Teaching Hospitals will apply for funds directly to the Minister of Health. Medical Schools will not be directly affected by the National Health Act.

Endowment Funds Are Pooled

Endowment capital of individual hospitals will be used for payment of indebtedness of individual hospitals, and the balance will be pooled in regional funds, the income of which may be allocated by the Regional Hospital Boards for such services as nursing education, training of hospital administrators, and medical research. All operating expenses and capital expansion will be financed with money received from the Minister. No hospital may conduct a public drive for operating expenses or capital needs, but voluntary gifts may be received by the Regional Board on behalf of individual institutions.

Two large central hospital endowment funds will not be taken over by the Minister of Health: the King Edward's Hospital fund of London (6,000,000 pounds), and the Nuffield Provincial Hospital Trust with headquarters in Oxford. These agencies may continue to receive legacies or gifts as endowment or for current distribution. Their programs will supplement the benefits of the National Health Act, by encouraging and financing research, education and experimentation.

All medical practitioners electing to serve under the Act (in hospitals or health centers) will be paid salaries commensurate with their classification, with vacation and retirement provisions. Consultants and specialists will be permitted to supplement their hospital salaries by private practice in their present offices. General practitioners have no choice. They must elect full-time salaries or be entirely excluded from the program. Benefits to patients under the Act must be received from participating practitioners, and must be performed in, or authorized by, a hospital or health center. Physicians or dentists will not be recompensed under the Act for services performed in their private offices.

Events Leading Up to the Action

The National Health Act was not unexpected. Nor was it entirely unwelcome to a medical profession which had been estopped from receiving remuneration for work in voluntary hospitals. The middle-class public had been accustomed to financing voluntary hospitals (for the other fellow) by charitable contributions, and receiving their own services in nursing homes and small proprietary hospitals, the only places where attending doctors were permitted to collect fees for hospitalized cases.

The voluntary hospitals of England were stifled by the inertia and tradition of their medical staffs and trustees. Voluntary contributions of service by the British medical profession, and of money by the well-to-do, sufficed until the first World War. Up to that time, hospitals had been avoided by the middle-class population and obstetrical deliveries and surgical operations were performed in private residences and doctors' offices. But increased use and rising costs of general hospitals placed a financial burden upon the contributors who did not use the hospitals, and upon physicians who could not collect fees for service in them.

In the early 1920's, voluntary hospitals began to establish Contributory Schemes for near-indigent workers (with $1250 or less annual wages) who thereby received two new benefits: freedom from a means-test when admitted for free care to a voluntary hospital; and a feeling that they, too, were philanthropic supporters of the hospitals. The element of insurance against a possible economic loss was absent, as was also the concept of the hospital as a public service rather than a "haven for the poor." The contributory "schemes" provided new funds for voluntary hospitals, but never exceeded 10 per cent of the income of voluntary hospitals.

By 1929, the need for general hospital facilities prompted Parliament to authorize local governments to transform County Council Homes for the aged and infirm into fully equipped general hospitals with full-time medical staffs, and to finance them from the local "rates." These institutions were open to the entire population, and patients able to do so were asked to pay as much as the average per-diem costs of the institution. County-Council hospitals were widely used by low-salaried employees, as contrasted with low-wage workers eligible for contributory schemes.

Self-supporting insurance plans for full-pay patients never received active support from English physicians or voluntary hospitals. A small number of "pay-beds" were constructed or assigned in metropolitan voluntary hospitals, but for the most part these hospitals relied on the free services of physicians and the charitable impulses of voluntary contributors. By 1946, the 161 voluntary hospitals in London received only 24 per cent from contributory schemes and patients occupying pay-beds. Endowment income, gifts, legacies, etc. failed by $6,500,000 of meeting the operating deficits of these institutions.

The Lesson for America

Good health service costs money. American hospitals are now forced to compete with industry for personal services and supplies. Our voluntary hospitals receive 85 per cent of their revenue from patients through individual fees or voluntary insurance. Most of the income of medical specialists in America is received for services performed in voluntary hospitals.

Our American voluntary hospitals are democratic institutions used by the people who support them. No revolutionary changes are necessary to assure their continuance. But *accelerated evolution* is required if the people, the hospitals, and the profession are to maintain a voluntary program of health service. Many more people must be enrolled in voluntary insurance plans for physicians' services. The present 7,000,000 members in medical plans should soon equal the 30,000,000 subscribers to Blue Cross Hospital Plans.

Hospital income from ward patients (other than insurance patients) in the Philadelphia area is scarcely $4.50 per day as compared with per-diem costs of $9.00 or more. Ward-patients and ward-days comprise half the service of our general hospitals. Obviously not all of these people are in need of charity. But many are unable to pay their bills after they become hospital patients, and, of course, tradition compels physicians to attend them "free."

Health insurance for physicians and hospital services in minimum accommodations would remove a heavy burden from the patients themselves, from charitable contributors, from attending physicians, and from the taxpayers. It would also avoid the necessity for government-controlled health insurance or a complete system of State medicine.

America's hospitals and medical profession will shape their own destiny. Our situation differs from that of England. But sickness costs are uncertain and uneven and the public is ready for any practical program which will permit the individual to place medical care in the family budget along with other necessities. Physicians and hospitals must provide the necessary leadership or accept it from others.

The many commercial health insurance companies in the United States have enrolled approximately the same number of policyholders as the membership of Blue Cross, Blue Shield, and other nonprofit health service programs. This article suggests standards which should be adopted if health care providers are to accept service contracts with commercial carriers. It is adapted from a paper presented at the educational seminar of the Bureau of Health and Accident Underwriters, New York, March 1953, and published in The Modern Hospital, *July 1953.*

Commercial Insurance

Group prepayment of hospital bills has completely transformed the revenue pattern of voluntary hospitals in America during the last twenty years. In the year 1952 more than $500,000,000 was paid to American hospitals by Blue Cross plans, and a substantial additional amount was received from commercial insurance carriers and other group prepayment organizations.

Hospitals and the insurance industry of America are greatly affected by the uncertainty of illness. Hospitals have been "insuring" service to the entire community in an unsystematic way for a long time. This situation gave rise to the sponsorship of nonprofit organizations for prepaying hospital bills, by which more of the responsibility was shifted to the general public and the employed population.

Hospital insurance is of interest to nonprofit voluntary hospitals. Government institutions are unaffected inasmuch as they are financed primarily from taxation and receive relatively few paying patients. Proprietary hospitals, on the other hand, assume little direct responsibility for rendering charity service.

Blue Cross and commercial insurance have undoubtedly upgraded many individuals to full-paying status, who would otherwise have been a financial burden to hospitals. There is grave doubt as to whether the voluntary hospital system of America would have survived up to the present time if the insurance principle had not been so widely applied to placing hospital care in the family budget along with other necessities.

Voluntary hospitals bear a unique relationship to Blue Cross community-sponsored prepayment organizations. But the nonprofit character of Blue Cross is not its most significant distinction from commercial insurance activity. Far more important is the service-contract relationship between Blue Cross and hospitals, and the widely available uniform type of hospital protection.

A service-contract arrangement is not, and should not be, a "cut price" operation. The American Hospital Association affirms the principle that hospitals should be reimbursed at full cost for all services provided under contract with third-party agencies, including Blue Cross plans, cooperatives, industrial firms, governmental agencies, or commercial carriers. The goal is difficult to achieve in every instance, but the purpose of the service-contract is unmistakable, namely, that third-party agencies should pay the full costs of the services provided by hospitals to their beneficiaries as a group.

Voluntary hospitals are not competitors of private enterprise. Their basic function is to bring necessary care to the public. Their special objective is to serve humanity, not to continue their own existence. Commercial insurance will serve the hospital system most effectively to the extent that it recognizes the needs of voluntary hospitals in caring for the general public.

A.H.A Set Standards

Approximately fifteen years ago the American Hospital Association adopted a set of "approval" standards, and authorized use of the "Blue Cross" for certain nonprofit, hospital-sponsored organizations that were developing throughout the United States. It may contribute to the orderly development of hospital service in the United States if some thought is now given to standards by which the effectiveness of commercial insurance can be appraised as a form of nongovernmental insurance protection.

The following policies and procedures are suggested as standards by which the values of commercial insurance protection can be measured from the point of view of the voluntary hospitals:

1. Uniform benefits for group policyholders throughout each community offered by all carriers. The wide variety of benefits has been a cause of confusion and misunderstanding between hospital admitting officers and the employees of group policyholders. If there were a limited number of types of group protection offered throughout a trading area, it would be possible for the hospitals to develop more convenient admission procedures for policyholders. It is very difficult to approve admissions for patients with 300 or 400 different contracts, numbers which are often found in a metropolitan area.

2. A type of premium schedule that would be attractive to large proportions of the population in a community. When premiums are graded strictly according to composition of a group of policyholders, it may be possible to establish attractive rates for "preferred" risks. In contrast the "bad" risks may be unable to pay the higher premiums necessary to cover their service. Accordingly, subscribers needing the most service become those with the least protection. As a result, they become an economic burden upon the voluntary hospitals.

3. A general policy of permitting policyholders to continue hospital protection during temporary periods of unemployment. Most commercial group policies provide for automatic cancellation of coverage when a worker changes employers. This loss of protection throws a burden on the hospital, because relatively few unemployed persons seek the individual protection available. The result of the cancellation of group protection is an increased demand for free and part-pay service from the hospitals.

4. An acceptable program of enrolling individuals and small employed groups for hospitalization benefits. From the standpoint of acceptability, premiums for individuals and small groups should not be substantially higher than for group protection of large numbers of beneficiaries. A special problem is the coverage of elderly persons who have retired and self-employed persons not eligible for group enrollment. Such individuals now comprise a high proportion of those on the "free lists" of voluntary hospitals.

5. A central clearing house for certifying paid-up status on a community basis, and for authorizing benefit payments directly to hospitals. There is wide variation in the procedures for approval of benefits on the part of insurance carriers. Likewise there are wide differences in various individual and group policies. In addition, it is often difficult to obtain individual authorization for assignment of benefits and for direct payment to hospitals. When these factors are combined, it becomes difficult for admitting officers to authorize credit to beneficiaries of individual or group policyholders.

6. More comprehensive protection against the cost of hospitalization, including coverage for chronic illness. Limited coverage policies often lead to misunderstandings about payments for the benefits which are excluded from the insurance policy. If the patient or insurance carrier does not pay the entire hospital bill, it remains the hospital's responsibility to provide the necessary care. It is of slight advantage to a hospital if the insurance policyholders are merely the people who would have paid their bills anyway. Comprehensive coverage tends to upgrade a larger portion of the population than does a limited form of protection.

7. *Operating methods by which a high proportion of the policyholders' premiums will be available for payments for services.* A carrier's expenditures for selling policies, certification of benefits, and general management are not available for the payment of hospital bills. The average family coverage contract becomes "active" every two or three years. Uniformity of contracts reduces the expenditures for certification and general administration. Experience indicates that total overhead costs for selling and servicing a uniform contract within a community need not exceed 10 per cent of premiums.

Competition Is Desirable

The readers of this article will observe that "nonprofit" organization is not included as an essential standard for the development of an orderly insurance program that will serve the needs of the public and voluntary hospitals of this country. Competition among the individual companies as to efficient operation is desirable. It can be relied upon to achieve maximum benefits to the voluntary hospitals and the public, provided the foregoing standards are taken into account in the planning of insurance protection.

Voluntary hospitals have always been an informal type of insurance system for bringing hospital care to the people. It is their special responsibility to achieve the proper distribution of services to those who are in need. To the extent that commercial insurance is adapted to the needs of the hospitals which furnish care to policyholders, it will contribute to the development of a nongovernmental health program for our nation.

Part Three

Health Care Finance and Planning

Comment

These selected papers by Rufus Rorem on hospital financing and planning display a distinctive, individual point of view that is as worthy of serious attention today as it was when originally presented one and two generations ago. The several elements of this point of view are confidence in the power of facts to persuade critics; a firm belief in voluntary philanthropic giving, voluntary nonprofit sponsorship of institutions, and voluntary cooperation among such institutions in the interest of the community; and a will to pursue efficiency in production through full utilization of specialized personnel and facilities.

Although it is the content of Rorem's writings that enlists our interest today, the style sustains it. The contemporary reader will appreciate the directness and clarity of Rorem's exposition—the simple words, the telling phrase, the close link between words and numbers. The venturesome writer may even attempt to emulate the homespun analogy. Rorem's writings are timeless because they are free of jargon.

Rorem is preoccupied with the short-term general hospital operating under voluntary, nonprofit auspices: today's community hospital. This hospital consists of people who perform a variety of related professional tasks. Its leading actors are the physicians who decide whom to admit and the type and quantity of services patients will receive. Rorem sees important differences between hospital patients and ordinary "customers," especially in their ability to exercise freedom of choice.

The hospital patient is uncertain about the occurrence and cost of illness; the provider—hospital or physician—is uncertain about his ability to collect the bill, since "by custom and by law" patients who cannot pay for care are not to be denied it. The solution to both uncertainties is health insurance, which also tends to increase the total funds available to pay for care. As for those without insurance, proper public policy calls for government to be responsible for recipients of public assistance and for philanthropy to pay for those unable or unwilling to buy insurance. The several sources of payment combine to defray total expenses.

In order that these funds be employed responsibly, health care must be produced efficiently. To Rorem, a highly useful vehicle for controlling expenditures within an institution is accounting, which should reflect the uniform recording, classifying, and reporting of transactions. Accounting, however, is not a useful tool for rate making. Rorem suggests that joint costs in the hospital be allocated according to ability to pay. He refers to the possibility of a two-part payment formula—one part for standby costs to be paid by the well and the other part for operating costs to be paid by the ill. Rorem is concerned that the omission of fixed charges such as depreciation understates the total cost of care. He is even more concerned about the implications of capital expenditures for subsequent operating costs. "It is not the first cost," he tells us, "it is the upkeep which creates most financial problems for hositals."

Other, hospital-specific, devices are available to promote efficient production within the hospital. Aimed at achieving full utilization of indivisible health care resources, these devices comprise a long list, including nursing units with private or semi-private rooms, improved scheduling, and increased use of the hospital by ambulatory patients.

Coordination of services among institutions also furthers efficiency. To Rorem coordination is the essential content of planning, to be conducted by a well-informed, objective, full-time professional staff who report to a governing board representing the community and acting in its interest. The assets of the staff are its technical skills, information about hospitals and the community, close contacts with the field, prudent judgment, and the power of facts and reasoned argument to persuade. A competent staff can measure a community's medical need, but not in a simple, numerical fashion. In one article Rorem cautions against putting "figures above facts." In the context of planning he observes, "Statistics cannot replace sound judgment in appraisal of medical care [needs]." Rorem has profound confidence in planning through voluntary coordination. He writes, "As a matter of history, more hospital programs have been saved through joint action and planning than by professional and financial competition."

Without doubt Rorem's style is a shining star to follow. It is always desirable to think clearly and speak plainly.

Rorem's view of accounting as a tool of control by management is as valid today as it was 50 years ago. Unfortunately, his expertise in accounting—unusual among economists—has not been heeded, and hospital accounting has been used as a basis for rate making. Rorem's suggestion that joint costs might be allocated in relation to ability to pay has been disregarded. Since neither he nor others have developed his ideas on a two-part payment formula, they remain unapplied. His writings do not distinguish between hospital cost calculated retrospectively and cost projected prospectively; there was no reason to think along these lines before Medicare and Medicaid were enacted in 1965.

Rorem believes that health insurance should pay both the hospital bill and the doctor bill, so that the two providers are not competing for the patient's dollar. Further, insurance should pay the entire bill if the uncertain cost of illness is to be eliminated. Rorem does not mention any possible effects of insurance on utilization. I do not know whether he has considered the possibility of moral hazard and dismissed it as negligible or has simply neglected it.

For Rorem medical need, though not a number, is a fact which can be ascertained by skilled professionals and is independent of any influence exerted by the sheer availability of providers. Yet it is equally noteworthy that Rorem always puts the physician at the center of decision making in health care. At present it is still a matter of controversy whether the physician can—and does—induce the consumer's demand for health care. The resolution of this controversy would have marked implications for public policy.

Rorem's view of planning as a coordinating activity at the community level, to be carried out largely by a small professional staff, has been implemented and tested through his own activities in Philadelphia and Pittsburgh. As a long-time participant in hospital planning in New York and a close observer of planning in other local areas, I can attest to the high levels of competence and creativity displayed by Rorem and his staff. These qualities are certainly necessary for effective health planning, though I am not so certain that they are sufficient, particularly when the vital interests of individual institutions and of the community diverge to such an extent that they cannot be reconciled.

Now and then Rorem nods. As an ardent proponent of action, he may promise more than prudent judgment would allow. He promises a saving of five percent in hospital expenditures from the adoption of uniform accounting and reporting, but offers no basis for the estimate. He also promises a saving of five percent from coordinated planning, but does not give its derivation. A modern student of evaluation knows how difficult it would be to test and prove such claims in the real world.

Rorem knows the hospital so well that when he leaves it he seems to be subject to error. The man who predicts correctly the closing of hospital schools of nursing and the increasing use of private patients for teaching turns out to be way off the mark in predicting a substantial reliance on atomic energy and a continuation of the doctor shortage. Both the correct guesses and the wrong ones indicate that while the study of the past may illuminate present trends, it is not a reliable basis for forecasting when underlying conditions change drastically. A man's work is best appreciated in relation to the problems that he faces and the information available to him and to his contemporaries; application of 20-20 hindsight is neither fair nor useful.

HERBERT E. KLARMAN

Readers of this article in the June 1931 issue of the Journal of Accountancy *were surprised to learn that governmental and nonprofit hospitals in the United States did not maintain plant ledgers and include interest and depreciation as costs of producing health care. I was also surprised when I observed this fact in my studies for the Committee on the Costs of Medical Care. The situation changed when large purchasers of health care agreed to recognize these items as reimbursable costs for services provided to their beneficiaries, such as Medicare, Blue Cross–Blue Shield, and other participants.*

Fixed Charges in Hospital Accounting

Hospital service is a business entailing a large capital investment, with resulting high overhead costs. This fact has often been lost sight of by hospital executives and trustees. Ninety-one per cent of the investment in plant and equipment has been provided without expectation of repayment or earnings on the amounts contributed. Consequently the pressure to render an accurate accounting for fixed assets of hospitals, and for the fixed charges entailed, has been more or less removed from hospital administrators and accountants.

The laymen unfamiliar with hospital management might well assume that hospitals consider accounting for capital investment an important phase of planning and operation. Yet most hospital reports give no explicit recognition to the fixed charges resulting from the capital investment, once the plant and equipment have been made available and placed in use. Depreciation accounts are consistently omitted from the records of tax-supported government hospitals and of those under the auspices of nonprofit associations, which secure their original capital and much of their current income from voluntary contributions. Governmental and nonprofit hospitals under independent church auspices represent more than ninety per cent of the value of hospital plant and equipment in the United States.

Hospital service involves two major types of expenses. These are (a) fixed charges, such as depreciation, insurance, interest, and taxes, which are involved whether or not hospital plant and equipment are utilized; and (b) operating costs, which are incurred only when a hospital is available for the care of patients. Some of the operating costs, such as those for heat, light, power, administration, and housekeeping, are affected mainly by the degree to which facilities are held in "readiness to serve" patients. They vary only slightly with the degree to which patients are served. Other operating costs, such as for food, laundry, and medical and surgical supplies, tend to vary almost in direct ratio to the amount of service rendered.

The standard cost unit of hospital service has for many years been the "patient day" (day of bed care), and the measure of the rate of production has been the "percentage of occupancy" of the hospital beds. In recent years, the use of the scientific equipment and apparatus—such as X-ray and chemical laboratories—in the treatment of outpatients has made the patient day less significant; but total patient days are still regarded as the best available measure of the amount of service rendered by a hospital.

Cost per patient day (per-capita cost, per-diem cost) could be regarded as an accurate measure of hospital efficiency, if all hospitals were to calculate this quantity according to the same formula. Unfortunately no uniformity is followed in hospital accounting. A few institutions include fixed charges in their calculations of cost; most of them do not. Some include newborn infants as patients; others do not. Some hospitals report fractional days before or after a certain hour as full days; others do not. Operating costs of hospitals for acute medical and surgical cases tend to range from four to six dollars per patient day, with others as low as $2.00 or as high as $10.00 per patient day, depending on the quality or the volume of service rendered. Usually hospital accountants do not add the fixed charges to the operating costs to determine the total cost per patient day; consequently their figures tend both to understate the total costs of hospital service and to obscure the advantages to be gained from a high degree of utilization.

The heavy capital investment in hospitals requires that administrators and accountants should give it recognition through the maintenance of plant ledgers and depreciation accounts. This practice would have two desirable effects: it would emphasize the importance of a high rate of production in the lowering of unit costs; it would remind hospital administrators that an omission of fixed charges from the costs of a hospital's services not only fails to give the real cost of the service, but also makes impossible the comparison of total costs of one hospital with those of another.

The following table is introduced to show the extent to which the fixed charges per patient day vary with the amount of capital investment per bed and with the degree to which the beds are occupied by patients. The investments per bed are typical of the variations existing in the hospital field. Some of the large state nervous and mental institutions represent investments per bed of less than $1,000, whereas a few elaborate "teaching" hospitals in the metropolitan areas approach $20,000. The occupancy rate of sixty per cent represents the average for the "general" hospitals of the country in 1929, and the rate of seventy-five per cent is the minimum at which hospital experts consider that best economies can be achieved.

FIXED CHARGES PER PATIENT DAY COMPUTED FOR
VARIOUS INVESTMENTS PER BED AND AT 60 AND
75 PER CENT OCCUPANCY OF HOSPITAL CAPACITY

| | Annual Fixed | Fixed Charges per Patient-Day | |
Investment per Bed	Charges per Bed	Occupancy 60 Per Cent	Occupancy 75 Per Cent
$ 2,000	$ 160	$0.73	$0.58
3,000	240	1.11	0.88
4,000	320	1.46	1.17
5,000	400	1.83	1.46
6,000	480	2.19	1.75
7,000	560	2.56	2.04
8,000	640	2.92	2.34
10,000	800	3.65	2.92
12,000	960	4.38	3.50
15,000	1,200	5.55	4.38

The annual fixed charges are computed as eight per cent of the total capital investment: five per cent allowance for interest and three per cent for depreciation. The depreciation is estimated as follows: two per cent on the value of the buildings, assumed to be seventy per cent of the total, and ten per cent on "equipment," assumed to be fifteen per cent of the total. Land is assumed to be fifteen per cent. These figures for depreciation are somewhat below those ordinarily recommended by hospital accountants. Taxes are omitted in arriving at figures for the table, inasmuch as most hospitals are exempt from taxation. Insurance also is omitted, for according to the custom of hospital accountants it is included among the operating costs.

The figures in the table show two facts clearly: first, that in the ordinary hospital the fixed charges are a substantial amount, exceeding fifty cents a day in the cheapest type of accommodations when occupied to seventy-five per cent capacity, and exceeding five dollars in the more expensive plant and equipment; second, that substantial reductions in the burden of fixed charges may be accomplished through increased utilization, even within such a narrow range as from sixty to seventy-five per cent of bed capacity.

The records and reports of hospitals which include no allowances for interest and depreciation draw a false picture of the costs of the hospital care rendered by them. In the case of nonprofit associations, it frequently happens that a philanthropist of a community has erected and equipped a hospital and presented it to the trustees free from all capital indebtedness. The services of hospital plant and equipment are not less valuable because they are paid for by philanthropists or from taxes. From the point of view of a community, depreciation on capital investment represents an actual expenditure for hospital service, even though it may not require monthly or annual cash disbursements. It is sometimes said that a hospital which utilizes plant and equipment on which there is no outstanding indebtedness can be operated at lower costs because it need not pay interest or repay the principal of the debt. Such a statement is equivalent to saying that it is cheaper to live in one's own house than in that of another, for, by so doing, one need not pay rent. The financial reports of "voluntary hospitals" in England, Canada, and Australia often show allowances for depreciation in the expense accounts, although the percentage of income received from patients of "voluntary hospitals" is ordinarily much less than is paid by the patients to nonprofit association hospitals in the United States.

The problems of some nonprofit hospitals have been similar to those encountered in ordinary business enterprises. One church hospital owns land and buildings which were valued at $2,211,086.51, as of December 31, 1928. Of this total, $487,896.07 represented appreciation through appraisal of the land and buildings purchased before the main hospital building was erected in 1927. There were outstanding $1,700,000 of seven per cent mortgage bonds—approximately the total outlay for the existing plant and equipment. The interest payments on the fixed indebtedness in 1928 amounted to $134,044.36 (including amortization of $12,581 bond discount granted at the time of issuing the bonds). In addition there were sinking-fund requirements for redemption of the bonds, which amounted to approximately $40,000.

The hospital, being in California, was also required to pay general property taxes amounting to $20,729.42 in 1928. The current cash requirements attendant upon the ownership of the plant and equipment by this hospital were approximately $200,000 a year. The adult bed capacity of this institution was 277, so that the interest and depreciation per annum for each bed (whether occupied or not) were more than $700. The average occupancy during 1928 was eighty-three per cent, so that the annual disbursements for interest and debt retirement exceeded $800 per occupied bed, more than two dollars per patient day of care. This hospital is not an expensive one regarded from the point of view of original cost of construction; it is not operated for the profit of the trustees; but it has been financed under such conditions that interest and depreciation on hospital capital investment must be recognized by its administration as actual costs of hospital care.

I have asked many hospital superintendents why their accountants were instructed to ignore depreciation and interest allowances in the hospital's financial records and reports. The replies have usually been one of the following: (a) "Such a procedure would swell the total costs of my hospital and make it appear in a bad light when contrasted with other hospitals which have relatively smaller investments or omit such items entirely"; or (b) "It is inappropriate for a nonprofit hospital administering donated funds to recover the full commercial cost of its services."

The first statement indicates a tendency to place figures above facts, and illustrates the need for an entire reconsideration of the concept of hospital costs. It is true that depreciation and interest are not usually factors over which a given hospital superintendent has had any control, and such items should be clearly set off from the other costs of hospital care in the preparation of reports. But there is no logical reason why they should be excluded entirely.

The second objection brings up for consideration two very important aspects of depreciation and interest. In the first place, allowances for the services of hospital capital do not necessarily mean that such amounts should be recovered through charges against patients served in the hospital. In fact, the purpose underlying this procedure might well be to exclude depreciation and interest in the setting of certain fees. In the second place, no allocation of the fixed charges of special hospital services can be made unless allowances for interest and depreciation have been estimated. There are cases in nonprofit hospitals where patients in private rooms, or those requiring X-ray service, pay fees which cover by a wide margin the most liberal estimates of their total costs. If it were understood that interest and depreciation were calculated in the establishment of such fees, patients might be made better satisfied with the rates they pay.

In conclusion, it may be stated that fixed charges, represented by depreciation and interest allowances, are economic costs of hospital service, even though they are often met by communities through taxation or voluntary contributions rather than from the fees charged to patients. Individual hospitals which are freed from the burden of recovering fixed charges from patients' fees or other current income are not thereby freed from responsibility for wise utilization of plant and equipment.

A careful estimate and report of the fixed charges annually involved in a hospital's services would provide the basis for comparing total costs of hospitalization in different institutions and would prevent confusion where some hospitals, because of no indebtedness, are not compelled to recognize such items. The general public, which in some way or another must pay both fixed charges and operating costs, would have a better understanding of hospital problems if the two classes of expenditures were clearly presented. Hospital superintendents would find data concerning fixed charges of great value when faced with the need of increasing the income from patients' fees. An accounting for fixed charges does not necessarily imply that they should be met proportionately by the patients cared for in a hospital. It does, however, make possible the apportionment of fixed charges. As a result, they may be borne by that part of the public most suitable to carry them, and not inadvertently laid upon persons or groups that should not be required to bear them.

The next work was greeted warmly by hospital administrators who felt that rising price levels, higher wage demands, and greater public expectations excused them from responsibility for increased costs of health services. They ordered more than 100,000 reprints of the August-September 1950 issue of American Economic Security, *a journal of the United States Chamber of Commerce. I based this article on my observations while serving as executive director of the Hospital Council of Philadelphia.*

Why Hospital Costs Have Risen

Total annual operating costs of hospital care in the United States are approximately $2.5 billion, as compared with less than $1 billion fifteen years ago. The national cost per inhabitant is now about $18 a year, of which approximately half is spent in nongovernment hospitals, financed, primarily, by the patients individually or through Blue Cross and insurance plans.

In 1949, more than twice as many patients (16.7 million) were hospitalized in the United States as in 1934, when there were 7.2 million admissions.

The ratio of total hospital costs remains at one percent of the national income, a proportion which has been maintained as long as national estimates have been available for study. Patient income and taxation are now financing higher percentages of the total costs, with private philanthropy increasing at a much slower rate than total expenditures for hospital care. Accordingly, there is great interest in the problems of institutional expenditures and their impact upon individual patients.

Institutional Costs

The traditional "cost units" in hospital care have been the "inpatient day" and the "outpatient visit," with most administrators striving for a high percentage of bed occupancy to reduce the per diem costs of their institutions. But a number of factors have worked against the achievement of lower inpatient costs per day. They include the following: increased price level for supplies and materials; increased salary and wage level; more complex and varied diagnostic and treatment procedures; more private and semiprivate services; shorter average length of stay; greater expenditures for nursing and medical education; deferred modernization of plant and equipment; and fluctuating percentage of occupancy and utilization.

Nationally, the average length of stay for nongovernment hospitals is about eight days for each admission. More work is being accomplished in a shorter period of time, with the result that per diem costs have risen nearly 100 percent during the past five years. For a group of 18 general hospitals in Philadelphia, the average per diem costs, uniformly calculated, were $7 in the year 1945 and $13 in 1949, exclusive of allowances for depreciation on buildings and permanent equipment.

Diagnosis and Treatment Now Predominant Function

The hospital is changing from a repository for bed cases to a center for medical diagnosis and treatment. Many hospital inpatients are up and about within a few days following a major surgical operation, an obstetrical delivery, or drastic medical treatment. Custodial service by nurses and institutional employees is being replaced by active medical treatment involving the use of expensive drugs and by intensive care from professional specialists. Convalescence now begins during the period of active medical care. The patient does not require a period of time to recover from the shock of his hospital experience.

The shift of emphasis from bed and board to diagnosis and treatment justifies a shift in the administrator's attention from the cost per day to the cost per admission. The significant product of a hospital is a group of recovered or improved patients, not a quantity of patient days of bed occupancy. The first week of hospital care has always been the most expensive financially and the most intensive professionally. It is possible to reduce per diem expenses by extending the average length of stay. But such an objective would not assure greater per diem revenue from patients, even if professionally justifiable. Moreover, the practice would ultimately lead to a demand for expanded plant and equipment, with expenditures for new construction and current maintenance. Advances in medical science which have hastened recovery have also been a long-run blessing to those who administer hospitals and receive care in them.

Measurement of Hospital Costs

In Philadelphia, the Hospital Council has for two and a half years been calculating a new "unit" for measuring the use of the bed facilities of its member hospitals. This unit is "admissions-per-bed-per-year," that is, the number of patients who have, on the average, used each of the hospital beds in a twelve-month period. In a very real sense, this may be regarded as the equivalent of merchandise turnover in a retail or wholesale establishment, which ratio is often regarded as evidence of efficient management on behalf of stockholders and customers. What better measure of the use of publicly provided hospital facilities than the number of different patients it has been able to serve during a period of time? In general hospitals, the range is from 24 to 36 admissions-per-bed-per-year.

A discussion of utilization and costs must include specific reference to the hospital's service to ambulatory patients who are not assigned beds for overnight residence. The character of outpatient service is changing. A decade ago, most patients were free cases seeking treatment for minor ailments which might otherwise have been treated in a doctor's private office. Now, a large number are private patients referred by physicians for diagnostic services which the private physician is unable personally to provide. Often the doctor will meet his private patient at the hospital for a consultation following a visit for diagnostic services in the institution.

The growth of private outpatient services has a profound effect upon costs to hospitals and costs to patients. The greater use of special facilities (radiology, pathology, physiotherapy, cardiography, etc.) reduces the costs of such services which need to be charged against inpatient care. Occasionally, such services to private physicians' cases may actually avoid the necessity of admission for overnight bed care. Thus the trend in hospital service reaches the superlative degree which has been sought by physicians for many years. The positive degree is "get people into hospitals." The comparative degree is "get them out of hospitals." The superlative degree is "keep them out of hospitals" by adequate prevention, diagnosis, and treatment while they are up and about.

The Patient's Problem

Hospital patients have always thought hospital bills were high, even in Philadelphia 35 years ago, when private rooms were priced at $3 a day "and up." The percentage of free admissions was higher in 1916, when ward rates were $1.50, than at present, when they average five or six times that amount.

Hospital patients are paying more money, with less complaint, than ever before. When private hospital bills averaged $5 a day, only a small percentage of patients paid the full costs. Now, when ward hospital bills average $12 a day, most patients expect to pay their hospital bill, or present a good reason for not doing so. A generation ago, people didn't bother to complain about the costs. They merely accepted the services free and complained about the food.

Why this change in point of view? In my opinion, it rests in the basic change in the public's attitude toward hospitalization. Thirty years ago, hospital service was essentially a charitable function provided by one group of the population for the benefit of another group, through taxation or voluntary philanthropy. The people who supported the hospitals financially were not the people who utilized their services. Patients able to afford hospital care studiously avoided hospitals, except for major surgical operations.

Patients Pay the Costs

The situation has changed. Now, almost anyone may be a hospital patient. On the average, each family will provide a hospital case every two or three years. The greater frequency of use has been accompanied by a rising price level for wages and supplies, without a proportionate increase in endowment income, voluntary contributions, or tax appropriations. The hospital gradually has been transformed from a charitable service for the poor to a self-supporting service for the entire population. The people who pay the bills are now the same people as the ones who receive the services.

Hospital costs have always been uncertain as far as individuals are concerned. The insurance principle has removed this hazard from self-supporting individuals, but hospital revenue has remained uncertain, because the noninusred population includes many people who are unable or unwilling to pay the full costs of the care they receive. The financial burden of their service must be borne by the insurance-protected group, the paying noncontract patients, the voluntary contributors, and the taxpayers. The greatest portion of the burden, thus far, has been carried by the individual private patients without Blue Cross or insurance protection.

The present high charges to private noncontract patients must be regarded as a temporary and unstable substitute for insurance protection, philanthropy, and taxation in the financing of free service to the people unable or unwilling to pay established fees for hospital care. It is a historical fact that governmental agencies have been reluctant to absorb the full costs of welfare services formerly provided (or neglected) by private philanthropy.

Attitude of Contract Subscribers

The large groups of contract subscribers have argued, not without merit, that they wish to finance their own care through their periodic payments, not the costs of service to their fellow workers who are too improvident to accept Blue Cross or insurance protection. They assert a willingness, as citizens, to pay taxes or contribute to community funds for service to the indigent or unemployed, but resist, along with individual full-pay noncontract patients, the hospitals' policy of making a surcharge on behalf of the other patients.

Is this attitude justified? The voluntary hospitals have no immediate alternative in their accepted program of serving all persons according to their medical needs. Assessment upon Blue Cross plans and private noncontract patients is the halfway point toward the final goals of enrolling all employed persons in prepayment plans, and the development of tax support for the unemployed and otherwise needy population. This fact makes it incumbent upon hospital trustees, management, and medical staffs to enroll the maximum number in prepayment plans, and to support long-run programs for governmental care of needy patients, and short-run plans for the financing of needy hospitals.

A hospital inpatient gets his money's worth in a well-run hospital, and especially at the present time. The shorter stay involves higher per diem charges, but, in many cases, a lower total fee than ten years ago. Moreover, the early discharge shortens the absence from gainful employment or the disruption of the household economy. In addition, it has become possible for paying patients to avail themselves of scientific apparatus and professional personnel, without permanent interruption of work. But until hospital costs can be placed in the family budget along with other necessities, including physicians' services, we may expect to find a certain amount of complaint about the costs of hospital care—for *even a reasonable price seems too high for something one does not wish to buy*. From the patient's point of view, a reasonable price for hospital service is a charge that has been adjusted to his ability to pay at the time of the illness.

Methods for Improved Administration

This essay is not intended as an apology for hospital costs at whatever level they may be incurred by a particular institution. The general use of hospitals imposes a special obligation upon trustees, management, and staff to provide the maximum service from the facilities and personnel. Some of the methods suggested for greater adoption by hospitals are summarized:

1. *Uniform accounting*, by which hospitals can compare the experiences of different departments and methods, as well as lay the foundations for comparison with each other. The insight into problems resulting from better accounting would, in the writer's opinion, achieve from 5 to 10 percent more service without increased costs. At 5 percent, the national saving would exceed $100 million annually.

2. *Encouragement of private outpatient service.* Diagnostic apparatus and professional personnel are seldom used to capacity in the service of bed cases or free outpatients. Individual medical practioners have welcome the opportunity to send private cases to hospitals for study and reports.

3. *Standardization and simplification of supplies.* There is convincing evidence that costs of institutional and professional supplies are higher than necessary, because of the expense placed upon manufacturers and wholesalers who must provide a wide variety of products for the same purposes.

4. *Group purchasing.* It is reasonable that economies can be achieved through large-scale purchasing, without sacrifice of quality or of service. Group buying is both a method and a point of view. It tends to make purchasing a scientific profession by group examination of the benefits of certain commodities, terms, standards, service, and price. No prerogatives are surrendered by purchasing agents, for their own agency must still compete with other sources of supply.

5. *Closer coordination between attending physicians and hospital management in the prescription of medical services for patients.* The medical staff influences both costs to the hospital and charges to the patients. There is evidence, in some institutions, that services have occasionally been prescribed, particularly for contract patients, which have involved undue expense to the hospital or patient. In some cases, the doctor has not realized the financial burden created by his decision.

6. *Coordination among hospitals in the use of professional equipment and personnel.* Not all hospitals should attempt to provide all types of diagnostic and treatment facilities. A high percentage of bed occupancy and a high degree of use of scientific apparatus are essential to low operating costs and acceptable charges to the public.

Hospital care is a professional and financial bargain. What does it profit a man to protect his bank account and endanger his life? Hospital costs have risen, from the standpoint of the nation, the institution, and the patient. But careful hospital administration can keep the total within a reasonable proportion of the national economy. Proper coordination of hospital care with medical service will achieve an effective distribution among the people who require service.

Originally presented November 11, 1953, at the eighty-first annual meeting of the American Public Health Association in New York City, with the title "Appraisal and Priority Standards for Community Hospital Surveys," this paper was published in the September 1954 issue of the American Journal of Public Health. *Twenty-two years later it was printed in the March 1976 issue of* Hospital Financial Management, *with the title "The More Things Change—Planning in 1930, 1954, and 1960." By that time I was retired from full-time professional activities.*

Standards and Priorities for Areawide Planning

"The Public should exercise better control over its capital investment in hospitals. . . . The quality of care is, of course, in the hands of physicians and the professions concerned with hospitalization. . . . But the public is entitled to control the expenditures. . . . Any community should view with alarm the expansion of hospital facilities except in response to a recognized immediate or future need." The foregoing statement from my book *The Public's Investment in Hospitals* (University of Chicago Press, 1930) referred to widespread activity in hospital construction during the preceding decade, when community coordination was not taken seriously. Times have changed—hospital planning is now a primary concern of local hospital bodies, philanthropic foundations, and governmental agencies.

Planning is not accomplished "in the abstract"; it involves daily actions by administrators, physicians, and trustees. Coordination among hospitals should have its counterpart in the program of each institution. Standards are the same for one hospital as for a group of them. Personnel and facilities must be utilized to conserve human and financial resources.

Expansion of hospital plant and equipment is not an unmixed blessing. New construction costs are inevitably followed by expenditures equal to 10 or 20 times the capital investment. These are necessary to finance service during the useful life of the buildings and equipment. After a community spends $2,000,000 to construct or expand a hospital, it must raise from $700,000 to $1,000,000 for annual operating expenses, assuming a constant price level and full utilization.

A community must anticipate trends in hospital service. These are more important than mileage data, hospital days per death, bed-death ratios, and beds per population. Six appraisal standards for community hospital surveys are submitted, which may serve as practical guides for programs of capital investment and current support. The article ends with four priority standards that appear justified in the light of modern trends in hospital service.

Appraisal Standards

1. *Evidence of unfilled public need for new facilities.* Plans for a single institution require data concerning all local hospitals and those in neighboring communities. Some potential contributors may not be interested in the expansion of a particular hospital. High occupancy at one hospital is not a convincing argument to an employer or group of workers who live and work in another part of the city, or to physicians who use other hospitals. A waiting list at one hospital does not necessarily justify expansion at the expense of the community. The writer recently surveyed a five-hospital city where the average bed occupancy ranged from 50 per cent to 95 per cent of available bed complement. At the peak of occupancy, there were more empty beds, in all hospitals combined, than the rated capacity of the largest hospital in the city.

A noticeable imbalance of bed utilization becomes a matter of concern to anyone who is asked to finance the expansion of a specific hospital. Some people will think or say, "Why don't the doctors and patients use the other institutions?" Trustees of one hospital may argue that it needs radium therapy apparatus because it is also available elsewhere, but a potential contributor may feel differently.

A community's needs may not always coincide with the ambitions of a single hospital's trustees or attending staff, or even the philanthropic preference of a large contributor. Institutional pride has been a great stimulus in many cities and population areas, but sooner or later someone must pay the total bill for hospital care. It is not the first cost, it is the upkeep which creates most financial problems for hospitals.

Idle plant and equipment are presumptive evidence that public needs have already been served, though the presumption may be wrong. Professional facilities and personnel may be overworked in some institutions, while expensive equipment and well-paid technicians elsewhere may be idle for large portions of each day or week. Data for measuring community needs include such facts as the following, applicable to several years: bed capacity of each institution, classified by beds per room and special limitations on their use; admissions and patient days per hospital, classified by accommodations, diagnoses, and seasonal variation; and checklists of diagnostic and treatment facilities at each institution, with monthly and annual data as to volume of professional services furnished for both inpatients and outpatients. There is need for objectivity in measuring community need, and the judgment of an "outsider" may be required to appraise the conflicting interests of local groups.

2. *Prospects for utilization of present and expanded facilities.* The public needs evidence to justify the prospects, and the "prospectus." Detailed questions arise: Have the waiting lists for elective hospitalization resulted from inflexible classification of room accommodations? Will medical, technical, and institutional staff become available to handle the enlarged program? What are the probable shifts in the proportions of private, semiprivate, and ward utilization? Does the change imply enlargement of the attending medical staff? If so, will the physicians merely transfer patients from other institutions? If the new program involves education or research activities, how will they affect staff privileges and the use of beds and treatment and diagnostic facilities?

The facts that provide answers to the foregoing questions are more difficult to obtain than statistics of patients, days, visits, procedures, and diagnoses. But much can be learned and predicted by an analysis of medical staff activity over a period of years. Significant data include number and type of staff appointments held by physicians at various hospitals; and number of inpatients admitted or served by each physician, classified by length of stay, type of accommodation occupied, pay status, and place of residence. Important also is the amount of time spent by each staff physician on the care of ambulatory patients and on the education program for doctors, nurses, and technicians, as well as the extent and character of his clinical, laboratory, or library research.

Measurement of effective use involves estimates of cost of construction and service. Hospital people often describe programs in terms of "investment per bed." Figures of $20,000 per bed are mentioned without apology, although a contributor may be impressed by the fact that his six-room suburban residence has just cost him a similar amount. Why, he may ask, does it require $20,000 worth of plant and equipment to serve him when he is hospitalized? One answer is, of course, that hospitals include much more than sleeping accommodations, which may occupy less than one-fourth of the hospital's total floor space. More significant is the cost of diagnostic and treatment apparatus for bed patients, as well as those who are up and about.

There is need to replace the term "investment per bed" with some expression more descriptive of the present functions of hospital plant and equipment. The investment might more properly be related to the total volume of service which will be performed during a year or the life of the institution. A 200-bed hospital may involve $4,000,000 capital investment (or more). Each year such a hospital would serve about 6,000 inpatients. It will probably admit 250,000 inpatients during 40 years of service to the community. These data yield an average of $16 investment per inpatient admission. The hospital will also serve many ambulatory patients, conduct educational programs, contribute to medical knowledge, as well as promote public health and education.

Bed occupancy data should be supplemented by more significant measures of hospital utilization. The Hospital Council of Philadelphia for the past seven years has calculated the average number of admissions per bed per year for each hospital. Statistics cannot replace sound judgment in appraisal of medical care, but history is a good foundation for prophecy. What a hospital has already accomplished indicates the direction and tempo of its future growth.

3. Physical depreciation or obsolescence of existing plant and equipment. Judgments on this subject involve engineering, medical, and administrative opinion. Nonfire-resistant facilities may endanger the lives or health of patients, employees, staff, or visitors. Improper design and layout may interfere with effective use of personnel and supplies, but these facts do not justify an irresponsible attitude toward the abandonment of present plant and equipment.

Prudence requires careful study of the costs and values of renovating or remodeling existing facilities. A renovated facility will normally have a shorter useful life than a new building or set of buildings. But a $100,000 expenditure may extend the useful life of a wing or building for 10 years. In contrast, complete replacement might entail $1,000,000 of investment. These are amounts of a different order of magnitude. Careful consideration should be given to alternative uses for the additional $900,000.

A structure that is unsatisfactory for one purpose might serve reasonably well for another. Patient pavilions have been transformed to employee residences, classrooms, outpatient services, or offices for private medical practioners. In Philadelphia, recently, a large general hospital, composed of buildings erected from 30 to 80 years ago, was purchased in its entirety by the Commonwealth for care of tuberculosis patients. The layout had become unsuitable for modern medical care of acutely ill patients. But the buildings will "last" another 50 years following various fireproofing procedures without basic structural changes.

It may be argued that all medical care in hospitals should be provided in modern buildings which reflect the most recent knowledge and skill in engineering and architecture. Obsolescence is a relative term, and must be used with respect to a program of professional service. Even the expression "fire-resistant" has been defined by safety and fire prevention agencies in terms of alternative services of an institution.

4. Relation to programs of other hospitals in the area. A hospital may serve the public best by supplementing rather than duplicating the program of another institution. Some hospitals have learned about other programs "the hard way." One institution approached a national concern for a contribution, using the argument that the firm had previously contributed to expansion of bed capacity at another hospital. The officers of the business were unimpressed because they had already relieved a shortage and saw no reason to encourage overbuilding. In another instance, a large enterprise had helped to finance an entirely new hospital near its new factory "across the river." When solicited by trustees of an existing hospital, representatives of the firm took the position that pressure had already been relieved from center-city institutions.

There is a tendency for each institution in a multiple-hospital area to feel completely responsible for all service to an expanding community. A recent survey of a six-hospital city revealed 900 available beds for a territory of 250,000 persons, with expected growth to 350,000 in 10 years. These institutions had drafted independent plans to build 600 more "beds." In addition, two new hospitals were under construction to provide 450 more beds in the "outlying" territory. When these facts were known, the trustees of one hospital shifted their plans to improvement of their present professional program without expansion of bed facilities.

Another example of the importance of knowledge of plans appeared in the projected expansion of a small special (orthopedic) hospital. Each of the community's voluntary general hospitals maintained an active orthopedic service similar in size and character to that in the special hospital. Moreover, each general hospital enjoyed the economic advantage of sharing overhead costs with other departments. As a result of the information made available, the trustees of the "special" hospital decided to consider merger or consolidation with one of the large general hospitals in the area.

Coordination is human as well as ideological. Some hospital people sincerely believe that survival is more important than economy or effective utilization. However, as a matter of history, more hospital programs have been saved through joint action and planning than by professional and financial competition.

5. *Prospects for financing current expenses which may result from the new capital expenditures.* Additional capital investment may "pay its way" by decreased payroll expenses or by improving quality of service, but ordinarily expanded facilities require additional income from patients, taxpayers, or voluntary contributors. Financial plans should include estimates of the effects of the new program on number of inpatients and outpatients, proportions of pay and "free" services, prospects of community and governmental support, and possibilities that additions to the attending staff will be necessary. Any well managed institution can expand its program of free service, if there need be no thought of finances. But "free" service to the patient is someone's financial responsibility.

One community hospital contemplated an enlarged physical medicine and rehabilitation program, to be financed by annual voluntary contributions. A preliminary investigation showed that several other organizations expected to continue their "piecemeal" free services to special categories of crippled and disabled persons. Conferences resulted in a plan of coordination of rehabilitation services, expenses, and financial support. The hospital provided physical and occupational therapy, with a program of evaluation and prognosis. Other agencies offered vocational counseling, special education, sheltered employment, and placement in industry. The result was a stable financial program for complete rehabilitation services.

A voluntary hospital has an obligation to arrange full-cost reimbursement for public welfare cases, particularly if there is no established fund which will yield endowment income or no approved plan of annual community giving to avoid the need of tax support. Conversely, a local government hospital should make clear how much of the operating expenses will be met from new taxes and what portion will be collected from individual patients and contractual payments by third-party agencies.

Civic agencies, such as community chests, hospital or welfare councils, departments of health, and chambers of commerce, face a challenge and opportunity to appraise the total costs of hospitalized illness and to develop support which will maintain standards and achieve equitable distribution of service among the population.

The cost of "free" service to patients has often been improperly described as a "deficit" in hospital operations, when in fact, the cost of free service in a well-managed hospital is merely the value of care provided on behalf of the general public, for which the people should expect to pay. A hospital is a professional institution, not a bank or financial agency. The public which desires hospital care should both demand a fair estimate of, and accept responsibility for, the income necessary to finance an expanded program. It is unfair to permit enthusiastic trustees or physicians to expand a hospital beyond its capacity to develop adequate current support. Perhaps the time has come for the federal government to provide less money for new construction and more for costs of operating community hospitals. A change in emphasis would have a desirable effect on the quality and distribution of medical care in hospitals.

6. Recognition of modern trends in medical practice. The main purpose of a hospital is good medical care. High quality medical service has been provided in outmoded plant and equipment, and vice versa. It is more important for a community to obtain efficient professional service than to enjoy the convenience of modern architecture. Some of the trends in medical practice which affect hospital construction are early ambulation for bed patients, expansion of ambulatory service, growth of physical medicine, housing the chronically ill, and service to the homebound.

Early ambulation has concentrated diagnosis and treatment into shorter periods. It has also affected the way patients and personnel spend their time. Many inpatients occupy bedrooms (not to mention their "beds") for relatively small portions of each day. Much of the time they are in libraries, sunporches, or the various departments for diagnosis and treatment. The bedroom portion of a hospital has tended to become a "dormitory," although few institutions have permitted patients to share a dining room at mealtime. Rooms arranged to serve horizontal patients for long periods are not necessarily suitable for short-stay patients who are up and about most of the time.

Physicians refer many private ambulatory patients to hospitals for laboratory tests and diagnostic work-ups. These private vertical patients should be received in adequate waiting rooms on an appointment basis, and the doctors should be provided with suitable space for consultations. This trend is a convenience to private physicians. It also permits effective use of the diagnostic and treatment facilities.

Ambulatory care at hospitals is more than a convenient device for handling emergencies in off-hours, and for reducing the overhead costs of a physician's service to nonpaying patients. It often provides prompt treatment, which makes it possible to avoid inpatient hospitalization.

The proper housing of long-stay patients in general hospitals deserves more consideration. Such cases are few in number and seldom require intensive service. But they account for a high percentage of patient days. Long-stay patients may be grouped in special portions of the hospital for custodial care. Hospitals often view with concern the occupancy of beds by patients no longer in need of intensive professional service.

Some prolonged illnesses, involving a severe physical handicap or disability, can be "upgraded" by physical medicine with a reduction in their hospital stay or an increase in the self-help. In the long run, even the active rehabilitation procedures reduce the medical needs and financial cost of institutional care.

Rehabilitation personnel and facilities are properly to be located in general hospitals, in order to assure contact with consultants in all medical specialites. There is a tendency for physical medicine departments to be assigned "leftover" space, made available through adaptations of heating facilities from coal to other fuel. New professional departments should be given equal consideration in renovation and new construction.

In passing, it may be mentioned that most new activities in hospitals were started in cast-off facilities. It is still common to find radiology and pathology departments in basements or far corners, not to mention the makeshift quarters for metabolism tests and cardiography. This "old-clothes-to-Sam" practice may continue for some time. The important thing is to recognize current practices in medical care and to plan capital expenditures in accord with observable trends.

Promise for effective use of capital investment is found in home care. The medical staff is assisted by visiting nurses and subordinate personnel or family members, without the expense of maintaining a bed in a general hospital. Consultants may be called to the bedside at home, or the patient may be transported to the hospital for special examination or treatment. Home care is a special form of hospital service, patients being merely further from the center of the hospital building. It exemplifies the fact that a hospital is "people at work," under the same supervision but not under the same roof. It carries to its logical conclusion the fact that the distinctive character of a hospital is medical service, not custodial care.

A hospital's staff, trustees, and management have an obligation to maximize the utilization of personnel and equipment by all possible means, including that of breaking with traditional practices. A patient sick at home is still in need of medical care which may exceed the knowledge, skill, and amount of time which an individual general practitioner can furnish. He can be a hospital patient medically, without the need of institutional care between professional visits.

Population data, patient days, and highway mileage are insufficient evidence to justify establishment of a new hospital, or even the expansion of facilities at an existing institution. More important considerations are, Will the professional care be of high standard? Will the facilities and personnel be utilized to a reasonable degree? Is the community prepared to finance the care which it expects to receive in the new or expanded institution? If the answer is "yes" to each of these questions, the trustees and attending staff of a hospital are justified in pressing their claims for capital expenditures upon their community.

Priority Standards

Though expansion of total bed facilities is not always the most pressing need of a community, capital replacement and expansion are inevitably required by the growth of population, the passage of time, progress in medical knowledge and skill, and new demands upon institutions to serve as centers for medical service, research, and education. The following priority standards are offered as a guide. It is assumed that "true medical need" might often exceed the active economic demand and also that available funds are limited. The sequence indicates the order of priority in capital expenditures. The basic consideration in these priorities is effective utilization of personnel and facilities. The viewpoint is that of the community.

1. Capital expenditures to achieve coordination among hospitals. Medical opinion is unanimous that a small hospital cannot provide a high standard of general medical service with a reasonable expenditure of time, energy, and money. A metropolitan area hospital should have at least 200 available beds if it is to furnish the major forms of diagnostic and treatment equipment, and diagnostic facilities must be used by vertical as well as horizontal patients if the hospital is to justify the employment of qualified technical personnel. Small cities and rural areas may be served by smaller hospitals, but in such cases it becomes even more important for the professional personnel and equipment to be available for the entire population, not merely those who require bed care.

The burden is upon a small hospital to prove that it will become large enough to provide complete care with reasonable economy. Plans by hospital trustees and staffs to coordinate their programs, even through informal agreements, should be encouraged. Examples may be joint housing of nursing school students, rental agreements for use of laundries or power plants, contractual arrangements for professional access to diagnostic equipment, joint purchasing agreements for staple supplies, areawide blood banks, development of central "premature" nurseries, interchange of personnel and respirators during polio epidemics, and joint use of rehabilitation centers for education and training.

2. Capital expenditures to increase utilization within hospitals. One example is the transformation of wards into semiprivate accommodations to achieve greater flexibility in the use of beds. Another is the provision of additional diagnostic and treatment facilities, particularly for ambulatory patients. Still another is the initiation of rehabilitation services for the disabled and chronically ill, ultimately reducing the community's demands for inpatient care.

Additional examples of capital investment that would coordinate the professional personnel and use of the publicly owned facilities are physicians' office buildings sponsored or owned by hospitals and adjacent to them (although ultimately they should be self-supporting); training programs (in so far as they involve investment) for submedical, technical, and institutional personnel; and experimentation with extramural services, such as home care programs for the chronically ill and housing of such public health services as may suitably be located in a hospital building.

3. Capital investment to prolong the useful life of plant and equipment. Many items of plant and equipment can be continued in public service by skillful renovation or remodeling. This does not imply approval of a penny-wise, patch-up policy which will reduce standards of care or merely conceal an actual need for replacement. However, renovation or remodeling may often extend the useful life of a building for a substantial period of time. It may improve the quality of medical care without a corresponding increase in operating costs. It may release valuable space for more important professional or institutional services, in the same hospital, in another hospital, or in a related area of public need.

4. Capital investment to increase bed facilities. Only when a community's needs cannot be served by coordination, renovation, remodeling, or replacement of existing facilities, should construction of a new hospital or the expansion of bed capacity be undertaken. This conservative statement may disappoint civic leaders or medical practitioners who have regarded the provision of more bed facilities as desirable under all circumstances, particularly in small towns or rural communities. A hospital is more than buildings and equipment. A hospital is an aggregate of professional persons in action. Unless their services are of high quality, and are utilized fully, a new or expanded hospital may give a community a false sense of security in its search for adequate medical care.

Conclusion

Hospital capital has always been provided by the general public, without expectation of repayment or earnings on the investment, and there is no prospect of change in this situation. Private donors, particularly business firms or foundations, tend to regard hospitals as instruments of public service rather than memorials to worthy citizens. Hospital sponsors must prove that the public's investment will be effectively utilized.

The capital invested in a hospital is not available for other forms of public service, such as a school, playground, or religious edifice. It cannot be recalled for some other important use. The character and degree of the need should be established before capital investment is authorized.

A hospital building commits future generations to finance the care received at the institution. A hospital's service program and financial requirements are not predictable beyond the most general limits, but capital investment affects professional policy for three or four decades. An error in employment of personnel can be promptly adjusted, but an unncessary building cannot lightly be dismissed.

Some residual value may lie in the possibility of overexpansion of general hospitals. Their capital campaigns are usually more successful than drives for facilities for mental illness, tuberculosis, rehabilitation, and care of the infirm aged. Entire "general" hospitals may become available for other aspects of health care.

This paper was prepared for a regional hospital association meeting when I was executive director of the Hospital Council of Philadelphia, Pennsylvania. It pointed out the multiple pricing system at institutions (full-pay, part-pay, and free) by which the "best" customers, commercially speaking, paid higher prices for services than the worst credit risks. It was published in the February 1958 issue of Hospital Accounting, *official journal of the Hospital Financial Management Association.*

Hospital Pricing: Theory and Practice

Hospital management and finance are often compared with private industry. The American people have invested more than 12 billion dollars in hospitals, and they pay in excess of 5.5 billion dollars annually for maintenance of the 7,000 institutions.

Hospitals Contrasted with Private Industry

But a hospital is more than a large business with extensive capital investment and complex problems of administration. A hospital is at once a hotel, a haven of refuge, and a program of life-giving service by devoted professional and institutional personnel. The management of a hospital requires understanding which is as broad and deep as life itself. It is complicated by the fact that each community expects its institutions to serve every person's need without regard to his ability to pay.

A hospital administrator faces difficulties which are not encountered in private industry. In business he needs merely to satisfy the customers which his firm selects, and the investors and creditors who contribute money, materials, or services through loans and investments. The social requirements of hospital administration must be thoroughly understood if practical solutions are to be found in the establishment and administration of a pricing policy for hospitals. This paper relates primarily to the "voluntary" hospital, that is, a nongovernmental, nonprofit institution.

In our government hospitals, very few patients pay (or are expected to pay) their hospital bills in full from their own resources. In sharp contrast, proprietary hospitals expect every patient to pay his bill in full, individually or through some third-party agency.

In private industry, the customer has an important voice in whether he will transact business with the vendor from whom he receives goods or services. He also determines the amount and type of goods or services which he will receive. These factors are absent from a hospital's transaction with its patients.

Hospitals Depart from the One-Price System

Pricing of hospital services was once a relatively simple problem. Most patients expected to have their bills paid by other persons, through the medium of philanthropy or taxation. A voluntary hospital was constructed by private philanthropy, and its current operation was financed by the same means. But the entire public now uses the institution. Most patients of voluntary hospitals meet the full costs of the services they receive. Some pay more than the costs.

Hospital economics departs from the "one-price" system followed by private enterprise. In a one-price system, all customers for a product in the same community pay the same price if they purchase in similar quantities and with identical terms of payment.

Nominally similar services are priced at different levels by hospitals in the same community. This is explained partly by the fact that the public considers—rightly or wrongly—that the services of different institutions have different economic values. From the point of view of classical economic theory, each hospital is a benevolent monopoly for a certain group of prospective customers. Needless to say, the attending staffs do not discourage this impression.

A hospital also charges individual patients different amounts for nominally similar services performed at the same institution. In private industry, the lowest prices are offered to the largest customers, who are often best able to pay. Lower hospital prices result from the patient's lack of ability to pay, rather than his knack for bargaining.

"Charity" discounts are not a phase of the "loss-leader" system used so widely in the retail business to attract customers for profit-making services or commodities. They represent a form of public assistance to certain members of the population. The hospital is providing care to public beneficiaries, for which the public should be expected to pay, directly or indirectly.

The fact that hospitals are expected to serve all emergency patients, without regard to their ability to reimburse the institution from their own resources, has complicated pricing policies for the voluntary hospitals, many of which have been forced to collect voluntary contributions from the well-to-do public, and to extract involuntary contributions from well-to-do patients.

Objectives of Hospital Pricing Policy

The objective of a voluntary hospital should be ultimately to make every patient a full-pay customer, with the necessary resources coming from the patient or his sponsors, or from the general public who pay taxes or make charitable contributions directly to the institutions. Well-to-do patients are typically careful purchasers of services or commodities. Many have objected to paying proportionately higher fees for the services they receive. It would be more logical, and probably more effective, if well-to-do patients were requested to make direct contributions at the time of their discharge from the hospital.

If hospitals were paid their established charges for all of their services, the matter of pricing would be greatly simplified. Four general purposes underlie the establishment of hospital charges.

1. The established charges should enable the institution to recover total expenses from those members of the public who benefit directly or indirectly. Actual patients benefit directly from the services they do receive. Potential patients benefit indirectly from the services they might receive. The institutions stand ready in case of emergency. Both operating costs and stand-by expenses must be met in some way, but not necessarily by the same methods.

2. The pricing policy should enable the institutions to maintain a high quality of professional and institutional care. Prices should not be so low as to depress standards of service, or so high as to limit utilization of the facilities.

3. The pricing policy should encourage an appropriate balance of professional and institutional service. Hospital stays should be as brief as possible, and the diagnostic and treatment services should be as complete as necessary.

4. Established charges should encourage the maximum use of hospital personnel and facilities. Idle time and idle equipment are a complete waste of professional knowledge and public investment.

Value vs. Cost Theory of Pricing

What is the basic theory upon which prices for services at hospitals should be established? In a competitive market, under a one-price system, there are two classic theories of price determination: the "value" theory and the "cost" theory. They are not mutually exclusive. In the short run, prices will not exceed the values placed upon economic goods by actual and potential customers; in the long run, prices will not fall below the costs of producing the goods or services, or of reproducing them.

Traditionally, the value theory has dominated the pricing of hospital services because many persons do not consider that different hospitals offer the same product; moreover, the individual's needs are imperative and require immediate fulfillment. During recent years, the cost theory has become more generally applicable. Scientific advances in medicine, specialized knowledge and skill, and the use of capital investment are factors in the change. Hospital service is more definable, and has become subject to the general operation of the law of supply and demand.

Depreciation as a Cost

If we agree that cost is the ultimate factor in pricing service at hospitals, let us consider the components of cost which affect hospital management and public policy, particularly some controversial items. Most frequently mentioned is the value of services of hospital plant and equipment, usually referred to as "depreciation." From the economic viewpoint, depreciation is as real a hospital cost as expenditures for salaries, food, fuel, or legal services. The only question is, who should pay this cost, or repay it?

Hospital patients are not the only persons to be considered in establishing charges for service, for the simple reason they are not the only people who benefit from the hospitals. *The hospital serves when it only stands and waits.* Ninety percent of the population do not receive hospital care during a given year. But a hospital is just as important for the 90 percent as for the 10 percent who are bed patients at the institution.

Logically, the readiness-to-serve costs (including depreciation) should be carried by the well people, and the operating costs met by those who become ill. But in any case, depreciation is an actual cost which must be paid by someone, whether a small number or a larger number of persons.

Depreciation is not always included in the accounting records of an institution, as one of the costs to be met through patients' fees. But it could be included. And it should be included in costs chargeable to any agency which represents a substantial portion of the public. Third-party prepayment agencies have an obligation (but no more than other patients) to contribute to the expansion and replacement of the hospitals of their community.

Interest as a Cost

An increasingly important item of hospital expense is the payment of interest upon borrowed capital for new construction, or for modernization and expansion of existing plant and equipment. Interest on borrowed capital is a legitimate business expense, and must ultimately be paid from some source. As far as the individual hospital is concerned, there can be no question that interest is an expense of operation.

A controversy arises when attempts are made to determine the responsibility of third-party agencies which have agreed to reimburse hospitals on the basis of the cost incurred for their beneficiaries. If a third-party agency reimburses one institution because it has incurred interest obligations to banking institutions or mortgage holders, should it also make a proportionate allowance to other institutions which have been foresighted or fortunate enough to obtain their capital investment from voluntary contributions? The answer to this question is to be determined by negotiations within a community. It will not be found in the accounting or economics textbooks.

As a matter of public policy, third-party agencies may well assume some responsibility for interest payments by community hospitals. But how about amortization of capital indebtedness? In my opinion this problem may be equitably solved by the simple device of depreciation allowances to each institution, which are sufficient to provide for ultimate replacement and modernization.

Problems of Cost Analysis

Hospitalization is a joint-cost industry. There are simultaneous and inseparable costs incurred in the production of the various services, such as board and room care, laboratories, operating rooms, outpatient clinics, etc. If any service is undertaken, expanded, or discontinued, it affects the cost and management of several others.

Shall board and room care be considered as the "main product" of the hospital, with outpatient service treated as a "by-product"? Shall each professional service be apportioned its share of the overhead cost, as well as those directly traceable to the type of service performed? For what units of service shall cost be determined? Shall cost be calcualted for each laboratory test, for each pharmaceutical prescription, for each

X-ray film, for each use of the operating room, for the preparation of a meal, for the use of a bed for a day?

In the writer's opinion, detailed cost information about each ancillary service is not significant for establishment of charges to patients. But costs for these departments may be calculated to serve an entirely different purpose. If the estimates are made in advance of expenditures, they become a very important guide to future policy. This is particularly true of "direct" expenses which are controllable by a responsible department head. The calculations are a suitable guide for the measurement of efficiency or trends in the cost of production.

From the patient's viewpoint, hospital service is a single experience. Very few of the services are performed because he wants them. He is more interested in the size than the composition of the hospital bill. It's not the cost, it's the uncertainty, which makes hospital bills so hard to pay and so difficult to collect. A pricing policy that will enable the patient to predict the amount of his bill will assist him in the payment of that bill.

Certainty vs. Freedom

Certainty is the factor which stabilizes hospital revenue under a plan of composite rates, including those paid through service contracts with Blue Cross and other third-party agencies. But the certainty is accompanied by certain limitations upon a hospital's freedom of action. In some cases, the computed cost of hospital service might be less than a well-to-do subscriber would have paid without insurance protection. To the extent that third-party agencies represent only well-to-do patients who would otherwise pay hospital bills from their personal resources, the contractual arrangements can be said to place a financial burden upon the hospitals.

Blue Cross plans and other third-party agencies argue, and very convincingly, that many of their subscribers would have found it impossible to pay established retail prices for services received at a hospital and would have been forced, otherwise, to request substantial discounts from regular charges. To the extent that hospital contracts upgrade the financial ability to pay of a group of patients, they can be said to remove a burden from the voluntary hospital, rather than add to others which already exist.

Hospital finance illustrates the paradox that low charges tend to increase hospital income from patients. A citizen has two alternatives with respect to hospital care when he considers hospital charges to be too high for him to pay. He can go without the necessary care, or he can go without paying for it. The result of high charges may be merely to increase the number of people who feel justified in asking for charity. This principle applies to prepayment subscribers, as well as individual patients. If the cost of protection against hospital bills is too high, or is thought to be, many people will attempt to receive care at the expense of the taxpayers or those who have joined health insurance programs.

Comprehensive Service as the Cost Unit

Comprehensive service is the cost unit of primary interest to individual patients and third-party agencies. Important problems of cost analysis must be solved. How much of the joint expenses of the institution are to be allocated to inpatient care and outpatient service, respectively? How are joint costs to be divided between board and room care and the ancillary professional services? What procedures are necessary to apportion the costs of ancillary services between inpatients and outpatients?

For board and room services the most significant unit is the "patient day." Diagnostic and treatment services to inpatients may also be computed in terms of patient days. For outpatient services the costs are more significantly computed in terms of visits, or actual procedures such as X-ray films, laboratory tests, etc.

Until recently, many hospitals established board and room charges at levels below the computed costs incurred for this service. In contrast, ancillary services have been typically priced at levels substantially above cost, including adequate reimbursement of all professional personnel. Board and room charges have increased in recent years, whereas ancillary service charges are about the same as they were ten years ago. *This is good for the people and good for the hospitals.* Higher charges for room service tend to encourage short stays. Lower charges for ancillary services tend to encourage good diagnosis and treatment. Some types of services might well be priced "below cost" to encourage their use.

General Applicability of Pricing Based on Cost

The basic principles for establishing charges for individual patients are not different from those for a group of patients for whom a third-party agency is responsible. In each case the charges should be related to the total cost of the services provided. For the individual patient, a summation of retail prices will represent the value of the services, provided they are based upon costs. For a third-party agency, the reasonableness of the payment is determined by whether it covers the proportionate share of the expenses incurred by the institution.

Calculation of the proportionate share is difficult, but not impossible. Are the third-party beneficiaries "average" patients, or do they receive an unusual amount or variety of service? Are the patients mainly people of average income, or do they include a high percentage of low-income individuals? Should cost be defined to include allowances for research, education and training programs? Should cost include an allowance for the costs of free service to noncontract patients?

The last mentioned factor is a matter of public policy rather than accounting technique. If hospital reimbursement for third-party beneficiaries is to include an allowance for free services to other patients, two conditions should be established. The third-party agency should receive explicit credit for this contribution to the health of the community, just as if it were paying taxes or contributing to a Community Chest campaign. Likewise, third-party payments for free services to other patients should be earmarked and paid to the institutions which actually provide the free care. They should not be distributed equally among the hospitals.

Summary and Conclusions

Cost of production should serve as the basis for establishing rates for services at hospitals. If an individual patient pays only part of his own bill, the balance should be furnished by the general public. Third-party agencies such as Blue Cross plans, insurance companies, or governmental agencies should likewise pay the full costs of the services which the hospitals provide to their beneficiaries. A hospital is a professional service institution—not a financial agency. The basis of reimbursement should be carefully defined in terms which are mutually satisfactory to the institution and the responsible parties.

Depreciation is an element of cost, no matter who pays the bill. Expansion, modernization, and replacement of plant are legitimate costs of hospital service, which must be paid by past, present, or future generations.

Certainty is important to both the hospital and the patient. Relatively low and predictable rates for services will encourage patients to pay their bills from their own resources.

The cost unit for establishing hospital charges should be as comprehensive as possible. This applies to both individual patients and to contracts with Blue Cross plans and other third-party agencies. The adequacy of payment to the hospital should be measured by the average cost per day, cost per case, or other unit of service.

It is desirable for hospitals to establish relatively high rates for board and room care, and relatively low rates for ancillary services. Ancillary services are the aspects of hospital care most essential to good diagnosis and treatment, yet least subject to control by the patient himself. Free access to ancillary services by private ambulatory patients would frequently release beds for other patients and emphasize the scientific and professional aspect of hospital care.

A price tag does not guarantee revenue. It often merely describes "what might have been." The pricing of individual services at hospitals should be determined with a view to the best possible balance of professional services on behalf of the patients.

A hospital does not give service in order to get money. But it must get money if it is going to give service. Proper study and consideration of costs will lead to appropriate balancing of institutional and professional services in the interest of better care for patients.

In 1962 I was invited to revise the article on hospitals for the forthcoming edition of the Encylopedia Britannica. *To my surprise I found that previous writers had not included a definition of the term "hospital," although they presented many significant facts and statistical data. Accordingly I developed the following definition, which appeared in the editions of 1963 through 1971: "HOSPITAL: A place equipped and staffed for diagnosis and treatment, where sick and injured persons receive medical care of such nature that some patients are required to use a bed during part or all of their stays. A hospital may be contrasted with a clinic or dispensary for ambulatory patients who return to their homes after each visit." If I were to revise the definition today, I would mention rehabilitation, home care, and preventive services as appropriate functions of a hospital.*

The following is a newspaper article which appeared in a special 175th anniversary issue (July 30, 1961) of the Pittsburgh Post Gazette. *A number of contributors wrote articles about their respective interests, and made predictions for the year 1986 when the publication would have existed for 200 years. At that time I was executive director of the Hospital Planning Association of Allegheny County. I suggested more than twenty ways in which hospitals would change during the next quarter-century, and the desk editor gave the article the headline "Hospitals of 1986 Will Be Used Less for Isolation and Custody and More as Service Centers for Ambulant Patients." The expectations have been exceeded during the past twenty years.*

The Hospital of 1986

By 1986, hospitals will change dramatically in appearance, scope of service, and method of financing. But a hospital will still be "people at work."

The essence of our nation's hospitals, 7,000 of them, is the knowledge and skill of 1,500,000 persons devoted to the prevention and care of sickness and injury.

Buildings, beds, and scientific apparatus are necessary. But they are merely instruments to assist physicians, nurses, and other hospital personnel in their work.

The total number of hospitals has not increased during the past 25 years. But they are larger and serve more people.

The modern hospital has changed from a place for isolation and custody to a comprehensive center for community health service. This trend will go still further.

In 1986, a patient walking into a hospital—and most hospital patients will walk in and walk out the same day—may be coming merely to see his personal physician who maintains a private office there. Or he may have been referred for laboratory tests, vocational advice, physical therapy, or psychiatric consultation. A small but important proportion of the hospital patients will be assigned to "beds" or required to stay overnight.

Patient-bed facilities occupy a small portion of a present-day community hospital's floor space—about 30 percent on the average. By 1986, this ratio will decrease to 20 percent or less.

Highly specialized operating rooms which resemble television studios, X-ray pathology, laboratories with electronic instruments and computing systems, social service, rehabilitation activities, psychiatric consultation, emergency care, outpatient services—all will occupy greatly expanded space in tomorrow's hospital.

Nursing education, public health, medical teaching and research, and doctors' offices will require larger areas.

The term "hospital patient" will be applied to many people who receive care from hospital personnel in their own homes, under "home-care" programs, or in separate convalescent facilities under the supervision of a general hospital and its professional personnel.

The shortage of doctors will be acute in 1986. An increasing number of practicing physicians will maintain private offices at hospitals in order to save time. This will apply particularly to surgeons, obstetricians, and other specialists who frequently use special diagnostic and therapeutic equipment and who "hospitalize" a substantial number of their patients.

The extent of professional change that will occur in hospitals between 1961 and 1986 is presaged by the fact that during each quarter-century the scope and power of the hospital life saving resources have expanded.

Each of the following facilities or techniques has been added to the general hospital armamentarium since 1936: artificial kidney, blood bank, bone bank, cobalt bomb, electroencephalograph, heart pacemaker, equipment for open-heart surgery, intravenous therapy, medical anesthesia, premature nurseries, radioisotopes, ultrasonic devices. There are others.

With rapid advances in medical research, it is safe to predict that the hospital of 1986 will contain an even greater number of diagnostic and treatment services unknown today.

Increasingly, the application of new medical discoveries will require the professional teamwork that is found only in a well-organized hospital.

New hospitals will be multi-story buildings, constructed to conserve

time and effort of professional and maintenance personnel. The overnight bed facilities, for the relatively few patients who require them,
will stress personal comfort and convenience.

Patients' rooms will contain no more than one or two beds, adjust-
able in height automatically. Semi-private beds will be separated by self-
operated movable partitions for privacy or companionship as desired.

Hospital costs will be higher. But the complaints will be fewer. Most
patients will not have to pay hospital bills when they are sick.

The bills will be paid in advance by the month, through some form
of group insurance such as Blue Cross or Blue Shield. The only out-
of-pocket expense will be for luxuries beyond medical necessity demanded by some patients.

"Uncle Sam" or the commonwealth or the local government will pay
for necessary services for patients unable or ineligible to participate in
group insurance plans. These will include the indigent, the unemployed, and certain categories of "retired" persons, also many of those
requiring long-term care, such as the mentally ill.

Some "downtown" metropolitan hospitals will merge. But this will
be offset by establishment of others in rapidly growing suburban areas.
The new hospitals will be one-stop health service-centers, offering a
wide range of professional services for both vertical and horizontal
patients.

The "size" of a hospital will be measured by the scope and variety
of its profesional services and facilities rather than the number of beds
available for overnight care.

Hospital programs and facilities will be expanded solely to fill unmet
community needs. Coordination and planning of total facilities will
become a standard procedure in all communities, following the example of New York City, Columbus, Chicago, Pittsburgh, Detroit, and
Los Angeles.

The management and medical staffs of different hospitals will cooperate actively in their health service programs.

Professional facilities of unusual types will be 'shared" by hospitals,
in the care of patients referred from other institutions.

"Visiting" at hospitals will decrease materially. On the one hand,
many hospital bed-patients will be discharged before their friends and
relatives realize they have been at the institution. On the other hand,
professional judgment will prevail over tradition, inasmuch as visitors
often retard rather than hasten a patient's recovery.

Parking facilities for visitors will become less important, but more
space will be needed for hourly parking by the many ambulatory patients who visit a hospital during each day.

As the hospital is used more widely by more people, hospitalization will be less of a conversation-piece.

Hospitals will benefit from advances in technology and management. Atomic energy will be used for heating or cooling portions or all of new buildings. Food will be electronically prepared, and stored in advance of delivery to patients' bedrooms or dining rooms.

Helicopters will replace ambulances or trucks when speed is required in transportation. Controlled television will be used in the supervision of patients and the instruction of professional personnel.

There will be many internal changes which do not affect the outward appearance of a hospital. For example, most patients will eat their meals in common dining rooms rather than individual bedrooms. Convalescent patients will wait on themselves much of the time.

Hospitals will cooperate with educational institutions in the training of professional nurses. General responsibility for nursing education will be assumed by colleges and universities with hospitals serving as facilities for professional experience and training.

This change is desirable. It will shift the economic burden of nursing education from the individual hospitals and their patients to the general community. There will be widespread development at hospitals of short-courses for inservice training of practical nurses, orderlies, aides, and attendants.

Private-duty nursing at hospitals will disappear. Patients requiring special professional care will be served by hospital-employed nurses, according to medical needs. The amount of "special" nursing for individual patients will be determined by the medical staff, not the patient's family or the size of his bank account.

Community hospitals will be used more widely for the education of interns and residents, and for post-graduate training of practicing physicians. They will also play an important role in clinical research.

Medical schools will not rely exclusively on "charity patients" for clinical instruction of medical students. Full-pay patients at "teaching" hospitals will be expected to participate in the educational program. Medical students will have an opportunity to observe the attitudes and viewpoints of private patients who will some day provide the major source of their professional incomes.

Hospital construction has been financed almost entirely by the general public, through voluntary contributions and government taxation. This will continue. But private philanthropy will place increasing emphasis upon teaching, research, and demonstration. Taxes will carry a large portion of the load for new facilities for patient care.

The total costs of health service will not decrease, even proportionately. As people grow older, they tend to have more sickness and less money. An older population will need to spend more for health services.

By 1986, we may spend seven or ten cents out of each dollar, instead of the present five percent of our gross national product.

Old age is the one chronic condition that everybody wants to prolong. By 1986, probably one-sixth of our population will have reached the age of 65 or older.

Before 1900, very few babies were born at hospitals. Since 1950, very few babies have been born elsewhere. At the turn of the century, a hospital was often the last stop before Sheol or paradise. But patients no longer abandon hope when they enter a hospital for professional services.

The function of the hospital has turned full cycle. Thirty years ago, the slogan was "get people into hospitals." The present watch word is "get people out of hospitals." The future requires that we "keep people out of hospitals," at least out of hospital beds.

The institution will provide within its walls a wide spectrum of preventive, diagnostic, treatment, and rehabilitation services, for both vertical and horizontal patients, and for both physical and mental illness. The hospital will also provide direction and supervision of services to home-bound patients, and to residents of nursing and convalescent homes for long-term illness.

The community general hospital has been transformed from a store house to a powerhouse for the provision of individual and community health services.

These comments represented my convictions after four and one-half years as executive director of the Hospital Planning Association of Allegheny County, Pennsylvania. On July 1, 1964, I "retired" to New York City where I worked for another five years as special consultant to the Health and Hospital Planning Council of Southern New York. This article was published in The Modern Hospital, *August 1964.*

Areawide Planning Is Here to Stay

Areawide planning is here to stay. The facts and the public interest demand it. Hospitals and other health facilities comprise an essential system of community service. They are not private competitive business enterprises.

For more than three decades attention has been called to the need for coordinating the economic development and administration of health services. Only in this way can maximum benefits be received from the public investment (through taxation and philanthropy) in buildings, equipment and personnel. Federal programs have recognized this need by requiring the various states to allocate Hill-Burton funds for new construction in accord with state hospital plans which designate community needs for health facilities.

Recent legislation has made certain Hill-Burton funds available for regional and areawide coordinated planning by nongovernment agencies established for the purpose. The goals and general activities of planning agencies may be mentioned briefly as background for the discussion of *auspices* and *areas* for coordination.

Detailed objectives of areawide planning may be grouped under the single purpose of *more effective use of a community's total health facilities and services, by the institutions, by the professions, and by the public.* Each institution's program affects the activities of all the others. Each health agency's plans affect the future of all other services in the community.

Areawide planning involves people and services. It is not accomplished by calculation of highway mileage or driving time, or by computing ratios of hospital beds to present or future population. Each health service institution must establish its own long-range plans for patient care (including prevention), for education, and for research. It is the function of an areawide planning agency to advise and coordinate the plans of all health institutions and personnel in the interest of the public who receive the care and pay the costs.

The guiding principles of coordinated planning may be stated as follows: Health facilities and services should be established solely in accord with proven unmet community needs; each facility or program should be developed in terms of a specific geographic area which may be shared with others; health care should be comprehensive and continuous, and may often involve joint action by service institutions; each health facility or program should provide sufficient volume of service to achieve quality and economy; the public should be kept fully informed about all existing or projected services and facilities.

The methods of applying these principles include such activities as continuous research through collection and analysis of health care statistics; frequent consultations with institutional and public representatives concerned with health facilities and services; development and coordination of long-range plans for individual agencies providing patient care, education, and research; public endorsement and recommendation of service programs and construction projects consistent with community needs.

These activities require the services of full-time professional staff concerned with the development and administration of health services, as well as sponsorship and support by public representatives.

Sponsorship of Planning

Who should sponsor areawide programs of coordinated planning for health facilities and services? The federal government has designated certain criteria for agencies which request financial support for community planning, which are briefly summarized in the following paragraphs.

The governing body should represent the general public, with the majority selected from civic leaders of demonstrated influence within the planning area.

Agency representatives should be authorized and willing to report their recommendations directly to the community, and to assist in implementation of approved plans and programs.

The community should be prepared to provide continuing financial support for an effective program administered by qualified professionals.

The coordinated planning should involve all types of health facilities and services, and be approved by and coordinated with the state Hill-Burton agency.

Some aspects of coordinated planning require active cooperation by practitioners and administrators. These involve such important matters as collection of statistics, joint accounting or purchasing, cooperative laundries or nursing schools, shared use of unusual professional equipment and personnel, public education, negotiations with governments and third-party payment agencies, and professional efforts to guide and influence the utilization of health insurance benefits and hospital services.

Decisions concerning the development or expansion of new facilities and services are properly the responsibility of the general public whose members will ultimately pay the bills for construction and maintenance. Actions should not be dependent solely upon the financial strength or professional prestige of a single institution.

The advice of health professionals is very important in matters affecting quality and cost of care. But professional counsel is most effective when the final responsibility is carried by persons not identified directly with any institution or professional group.

In Allegheny County, Pennsylvania, the Hospital Administrator's Advisory Committee has made specific recommendations on all applications for approval of programs or construction projects presented to the citizen-sponsorship Hospital Planning Association. It studies and discusses each application carefully with representatives of the institution seeking approval, and with other agencies which are most likely to be affected favorably or unfavorably.

Over a period of four and a half years, the trustees have followed the administrator's recommendation in every instance. In all but one case, the applicant institution was able to satisfy the committee that its program was consistent with a coordinated plan for Allegheny County, although usually this required some modification, reduction, addition, or deferral of the original proposal.

There can be no categorical inclusion or exclusion of individuals or groups on the governing body of an areawide planning agency. It is essential, however, that each director or trustee serve as a representative of the general public, whether he be an industrial or mercantile executive, a holder of public office, a labor union official, a welfare agency or hospital administrator, a practicing physician, dentist or nurse, a Blue Cross or insurance representative, a foundation executive, or chosen from some other field of activity.

There is no basic conflict between nongovernmental and governmental interest in areawide planning. Nongovernmental hospitals have for many years been affected by licensure and inspection programs, by governmental purchase of services to indigent persons, and Hill-Burton contributions under the annual state hospital plans throughout the country. There is no present Chinese Wall between governmental and nongovernmental health service and financing.

Governmental action does not lend itself naturally to a program of inspiration and leadership in health service. Equity requires establishment and enforcement of uniform administrative regulations. Licensure and inspection tend to stress minimum standards rather than ideal professional goals. Distribution of capital funds may be affected by differences in financial strength rather than professional standards of institutions.

Suitable Planning Area

There can be no single standard for determining the population or geographic area suitable for effective planning. Even a single-hospital county or city may serve the public and the institution by making a careful study and appraisal of present and future community needs. Conversely, a metroplitan planning area might properly include cities and counties in adjoining states.

An areawide planning agency should serve a population large enough to justify employment of full-time professional staff. Such an "area" should include a "core city" which also serves as the natural center of industrial, commercial, recreation, educational, welfare, and health services of neighboring communities. The character of the services offered by a planning agency will be affected by the frequency and intimacy of contacts with health institutions and the public representatives in all sections of the planning area.

For sustained advisory services by the professional staff, a radius of 50 or 75 miles might be considered the desirable limit for areawide planning. But if active long-range planning committees are established at each hospital or outlying community, the association may function effectively at considerable distance from a central headquarters.

Areawide planning is most effective when the public and institutions have a sense of identification with the community which is being served. A state-wide planning agency (except in the headquarters community), might expect to serve primarily as a coordinator for local planning councils in a number of small communities.

Coordinated planning may be applied to large or small population areas, but one million appears to be the minimum size to justify the full-time services of professional staff members with various types of training and experience.

Areawide planning can be most effective when it considers both public and private health facilities. These include general and special hospitals, nursing homes, old-folks homes, visiting nurse associations, home-care programs, rehabilitation centers, and child-guidance clinics. The coordination process is applicable among similar institutions, also among different types of services.

There are certain aspects which sharply differentiate a modern general hospital from other health agencies within a community, many of which have traditionally received substantial philanthropic support from United Funds or individual contributions. The capital investment and annual expenditures of a single general hospital may exceed the total of all the various United Fund (or Community Chest) health agencies combined.

Most general hospitals receive relatively small proportions of their income from individual or group contributions. Their health programs are established to provide a high quality of service at reasonable cost to all economic segments of the population.

Areawide planning costs money. Who should finance such an effort? The primary responsibility should be carried by the primary beneficiaries, namely, the general public who construct, who utilize, and who finance the institutional operations.

The hospital and health agencies discharge their responsibility simply by cooperating with each other to achieve efficiency and professional standards. Any payments by a hospital or health agency should be made solely for specific services rendered on behalf of a single institution or group of them.

How much should a community spend annually on coordinated planning for hospitals and related health services? It seems reasonable to expect that more cooperation and less duplication would make it possible to provide five percent more service and at no more expense to the community.

A community might properly spend at least one-tenth of one percent, or one mill per dollar of annual expenditures for areawide coordination. For a community of one million persons, this would be $60,000 annually, in contrast to $60 million for total operating expenses.

At $30,000 cost per new general hospital bed, coordinated planning effort for a population of one million persons would be justified if it resulted in the avoidance, deferral, or reduction of only *two* hospital beds per year. Several planning associations have been able to direct millions of dollars annually into more productive channels through their continued efforts in coordinated planning.

The community welfare requires that our vast public investment in health facilities and personnel be utilized effectively. This goal can only be achieved through coordinated planning by public representatives with the advice and counsel of health institutions and professions. The organization and method will change along with both knowledge and experience.

Facts, conviction, and action are essential to an effective program. The most important is action, which derives from a conviction that coordination will yield the greatest good for the greatest number.

This survey of capital needs and financing methods was published in the October 16, 1968 issue of Hospitals. *It shows that capital needs have changed from the addition of bed capacity in institutions and areas to accommodations for special diagnostic procedures and other services which can be more effectively provided on an ambulatory basis. Sources-of-funds information indicated that capital is increasingly provided through governmental loans, reimbursement allowances for interest and depreciation, and the sale of stocks or bonds to private investors.*

Changing Capital Needs and Financing

The first nationwide inquiry into the costs of health service began during the 1920s, a period of unprecedented affluence. The inquiry was conducted by the Committee on the Costs of Medical Care, a non-governmental research group established in 1928 and supported by private foundations. There was little or no unemployment. Wages were high. Investments were rising in value. The stock market crash was still to come. Medical care was improving in quality.

Total health care costs in 1929 represented only four percent of the gross national product. But there was a general conviction that the benefits of modern medicine were not reaching the people in a manner consistent with individual need and ability to pay.

The national studies revealed findings that were so universal and self-evident that they needed only to be stated to be accepted. Foremost was the fact that no one can foretell or control when he will be sick or injured, or what his illness or injury will cost him.

The second general fact was the degree to which health resources had been provided by the general public without expectation of financial return to those providing the capital investment. Even in 1928 more than 90 percent of the capital investment in hospital plant and equipment was located in governmental and nonprofit voluntary hospitals.

Investment and Cost

The custodial functions of hospitals once made it appropriate to measure facilities in terms of "investment per bed" and services in terms of "cost per patient day." But these units are becoming irrelevant to problems of management and the financing of health care. The facilities and functions that can properly be expressed in these units are decreasing in proportion to increases in financial investment, costs, and income.

The floor space of patient rooms in a typical general hospital is less than 25 percent of the total square footage of the institution. The rest of the space is used for operating rooms, dietary services, plant operation, laboratories, administration, employee accommodations, ambulatory care, and professional education and research. A bed is only one possible unit for expressing the degree of capital investment. Total investment per bed in a hospital is almost as inappropriate a concept as investment per window in an office building.

The same irrelevance applies to the unit known as "cost per patient day" in measuring health care expenditures. Differences in per diem costs result from many factors, including number and varieties of special facilities, qualifications of personnel, types of cases accepted for care (for example, young or old, acute or chronic, surgical or medical), building layout and design, degree of utilization (other facilities as well as beds) administrative effectiveness, areawide price levels, and managerial efficiency.

Capital Cost Reimbursement

Much time, worry, and study have been spent in search for the proper elements of reimbursable costs. Such determination is concerned basically with public policy rather than accounting procedures or marketplace pricing. It is essential to specify which segments of the public are to be responsible for financing each portion of a hospital's expenditures. Also, it should be determined whether, and to what degree, one group of patients should finance services to another group—specifically, whether the costs of "free" services to the needy should be included in the formula for reimbursement by third-party agencies.

Capital costs (interest, amortization, depreciation, and replacement allowances) are important in determining the adequacy of amounts paid to a hospital. If the purpose of capital cost allowances is merely to restore the original investment, what provision should be made to provide facilities in the future?

The book values appearing in the plant ledgers of hospitals tend to be substantially lower than the replacement costs of the buildings and equipment. Such understatement does not result from failure to apply normal accounting methods. Additions to recorded capital investment are made from time to time at different price levels. But the cost of replacement would be considerably higher than the original cost for a part of an institution constructed 10, 20, 30 or 40 years earlier. Even when facilities are appraised for insurance or other purposes, the new evaluations are seldom recorded in the double-entry records of the institution.

The United States government presently is concerned with "incentives" that will induce health care institutions to economize in spending the public's money, providing rewards (presumably monetary) for prudence, efficiency, and compassion in the care of individual patients. But it is doubtful whether this rainbow is attainable, unless the public approves in advance the organization and operating policies of hospitals.

It is imperative that financing agencies stop writing checks for past services and begin supporting future health care programs. If an institution wishes to initiate, expand, or discontinue a health program, its self-interest lies in adapting the program to the needs, wishes, and resources of the consumers of its services.

Capital cost allowances should be related to future capital requirements, not to the original cost of existing facilities. Few health care facilities would ever be replaced with the same layout and design. The construction costs would be affected by price and wage levels. Layout and design would be influenced by trends in medical practice and architecture.

It would be impossible for allowances for future capital needs to be paid currently to individual institutions. Allowances accumulated on the basis of a hospital's own services seldom would be adequate to finance a major capital expenditure. If the general public is to approve the need and provide the money for construction projects, sound policy suggests payment of total capital allowances into a central fund (after all, it's the public's money) to be drawn upon as each health care project receives public endorsement.

Capital cost allowances by government agencies represent a shift from governmental subsidy of institutions to governmental purchase of service from institutions. Reimbursement formulas ultimately are planning devices in spite of all arguments to the contrary. If the formulas do not include capital cost allowances, the public must later finance capital projects by intermittent taxation, philanthropy, or private investment.

Needs Have Changed

Major capital expenditures are infrequent and intermittent. A building remains in service for 30 to 40 years, even longer. Its replacement requires that special community effort provide philanthropic gifts or authorize necessary taxes and that institutions arrange commercial loans or provide investment. Spasmodic fund raising was reasonably effective at a time when hospitals and health facilities were in short supply. All additions to the number of hospitals and bed supply were desirable.

Capital needs have changed. There probably are enough hospitals in the nation, although some should be relocated for the convenience of the public and the health care professions. Bed capacity and utilization have remained static for several years. But increasing sums are being spent for modernization of plant and equipment to meet the increasing demand for outpatient services, extended care for the elderly, and other services precipitated by advances in technology and changing patient demands.

Although an institution's needs are intermittent and infrequent, a community's capital needs are regular and continuous. Moreover, the total community needs can be predicted from year to year.

Private and public health insurance programs, coupled with government purchasing of service for the needy, are becoming the major source of funds for hospital capital projects. Taxes, subscriptions, and premiums are forms of community health care financing that now provide approximately 80 percent of hospital revenue in the United States. This fact explains the increasing concern by third-party agencies for community planning of health care facilities.

Predictions

Capital needs and financing methods have changed materially in recent decades, but the past is merely prologue. The public will still provide the money for plant and equipment, but there will be new forms of public representation. For many years, general taxation and philanthropy carried the major responsibility, with minor participation through private investment and commercial loans.

The general public now expresses its will through 150 million Blue Cross subscribers and private health insurance policyholders. Another 20 million Medicare participants are represented by the federal government. Still others receive tax-supported care purchased from private or public institutions. Third-party payments to hospitals now are computed to include allowances for capital needs, whether based on costs of production or on prices determined by the institutions.

The following predictions appear reasonable in the light of observable trends in financing methods for hospital capital.

The number of hospitals in the United States will increase very little in the future. Some will be relocated, some will be merged, and others will be discontinued. The resulting institutions will be relatively large community health service centers.

Bed capacity will decrease in importance as a measure of the size of a hospital. Other standards will be number of ambulatory patients and visits, volume and variety of diagnostic and treatment procedures, programs for home care, facilities for long-term service, amount of money expended per year, and number of people served during a fiscal period.

Capital financing will become more regular and stabilized. This will be accomplished by the inclusion of allowances for replacement of plant and equipment in the prices and payments for health services at hospitals. The capital funds will still be provided by the general public, but increasingly as a "built-in" portion of the payments for comprehensive health services by public and private third-party agencies.

Hospitals will cooperate to a greater degree in sharing of certain services. Examples are purchasing, food service, accounting, data processing, central supply, and laundry. Unusual professional services will be concentrated in the larger institutions.

Community planning for new health facilities will develop from community financing programs for health care. Reimbursement for capital replacement relates to future needs, not past expenditures. Agreement to finance new construction implies the right to appraise and approve new projects and programs.

Philanthropy will continue to support and influence capital financing. But private or organized philanthropy may be expected to be selective in its financing policies. Of special interest will be the fields of research, education, and experimentation.

Hospital services will be more broadly defined. Patient care will include the functions of prevention, diagnosis, and rehabilitation. Education and research will be major purposes of the hospitals. Progressive care programs will adapt personnel and facilities to patient requirements for intensive service, continuing care, and self-help. Extramural services will include coordination with nursing homes and organized home care before, after, or in place of inpatient bed care.

I was invited to contribute a chapter on health care economics to a book entitled Depth and Extent of the Geriatric Problem, *published in 1970 by Charles C. Thomas, Inc. I find that the older we get the more care we need and the less money we have. There is no elderly way to suffer illness or disability, to remove an appendix, or to pay a hospital bill. The chapter is essentially a monograph on health care economics, with emphasis on problems of elderly persons.*

The Economics of Geriatric Health Care

We all hope to grow old; at least we hope to grow older. Every year more of us accomplish this objective. The birth rate has been going down, but the survival rate has been going up.

Older persons constitute both a resource and a responsibility for society. The resource consists of knowledge and experience concerning problems of living and making a living, albeit more often honored by neglect than recognition. The responsibility is to incorporate elderly persons into the mainstream of family and community living. They should participate in the production, distribution, and enjoyment of services and commodities, including the prevention of disability and the pursuit of health.

Health needs have many aspects—personal and social—which must be taken into consideration by individuals and groups. This essay will limit itself to those phases of health service which can be measured and discussed in financial terms. Health service costs money, and good health service costs a good deal of money. The financing of health service for the aged and aging utilizes the same methods as care for the general population. Someone must pay the bills. Who should pay, and how, and what effect do the methods have upon the quality of care and the equity of its distribution to those in need?

Special Economic Facts Concerning Health Needs of the Elderly

Old people, on the average, have less money than younger groups, except infants and dependent children. They have fewer assets and less current income for family maintenance.

The explanation is not difficult. Old age implies nonemployment or semiretirement. To be sure, there are many sexagenerians with retirement allowances and/or earnings which are sufficient to maintain a comfortable level of existence. But statistical studies of incomes all show that people over 65, who comprise only 10 percent of the population, account for 20 percent of those who are at the bottom of the income groupings. The legal maximum of old age social insurance benefits is a low percentage of one's previous earnings.

Studies have shown that many elderly persons have enough money to meet the costs of one surgical operation. But they also reveal that such payment affects the patient's ability to pay for food, clothing, and shelter.

No investigators have asserted that the average income for a group was assurance that any particular individual would be able to pay for necessary medical care from his own resources. It is recognized, if not expressed, that an individual's needs may be greater than the average needs for a group; also that an individual's income might not "come up to the average."

Even if statistical studies did not reveal that old people had relatively low average incomes, common sense and observation would compel one to reach the same conclusion. Most elderly persons have been retired, or fired. A large number suffer from disabilities which may have led to their unemployment. The over-65 people are predominantly women, most of whom were never in the labor market and have relied upon the earnings of their former husbands.

All studies lead to the same conclusion. The over-65 population have less money with which to pay for economic goods and services, including health care. Much study could have been avoided in social planning if this fact could have been posited as the basis for solutions of the problems. We do not need accurate statistical estimates to prove that one can not pay bills without money.

Health Service Needs of the Aged

Needs for health service tend to vary directly with the age of individuals and groups. The older we get the less money we have, and the more health care we need.

These facts are enough to establish the need for community financing of health care for the aged. The services must be financed by current earnings of the employed population, not the unemployed or the former employed. This situation prompted the recent Medicare legislation, by which health service benefits were added to the provisions of the old age and survivors' insurance program.

Before discussing the advantages and limitations of the new Medicare program, it is appropriate to document the assertion that the elderly population has needed, and received, proportionately more health service, on the average, than the rest of the population. The existence of need would appear to be self-evident. Older persons have acquired more varieties of disability, for the simple reason that they have lived longer. The older bodies require more attention to maintenance and repair, and are less able to resist infection or return to normalcy after an injury or period of sickness.

Older people have been receiving more total care, on the average, than the rest of the population. Old folks are hospitalized more often for medical and surgical conditions, and they stay in the general hospitals about twice as long as the other patients. They see a doctor more frequently than younger persons—at a physician's office, in a hospital outpatient department, or in their own homes. They comprise almost the total bed-population of nursing homes.

Elderly persons who are admitted to general hospitals receive more professional nursing care than other patients. Professor John D. Thompson and others at Yale University conducted a special study of the time devoted to nursing care of individual patients at fifty-five hospitals in nine cities in eight states during the year 1965. The study revealed that over-65 patients received an average of 4.97 hours of nursing care per patient day as compared to 4.06 hours for other medical and surgical patients. These figures apply to the time spent in direct patient contact by nurses, indirect professional services, and general functions not related to nursing.

The high demand for hospital bed care among elderly subscribers was of great concern to Blue Cross plans before the advent of Medicare. Subscribers over 65 years of age used three times as many patient days of hospitalization per subscriber as the rest of the enrolled population. The elder subscribers created a financial burden which had to be carried by the rest of the group. Arithmetically speaking, the plans could have afforded to pay a bonus to each elderly person who decided not to enroll.

Elderly people need large amounts of dental care, most of which is never received. Statistical studies show that expenditures for dental services are directly related to personal income rather than personal need for service. Much dentistry for the general population is of a nonemergency nature in the sense that it does not involve conditions which immediately endanger life or general health. But among elderly persons, dental needs may be directly related to personal health and well-being.

Most health insurance programs, including Medicare, limit dentistry benefits to emergency services involving traumatic conditions which require hospitalization or surgical procedures. Elective dental services are usually excluded because of the general assumption that they are subject to individual desires and therefore cannot be regarded as insurable risks. But the problem of financing dental care for older persons requires effective solution, and such benefits should be provided.

Geriatrics and the Family

Elder care is a family affair. Eighty per cent of all persons over 65 years of age have at least one living relative (spouse, sibling, child, or grandchild). And many others have close family ties.

What is the economic significance of the family in health care for the aged? Several points may be mentioned. First of all, the dividing line between good health and ill health is not sharply drawn in the case of elderly persons. Old age is itself a disability—a form of ill health. It is not self-limiting. One doesn't get over it, and he doesn't want to. There is no preferred alternative to growing older.

An elderly person is like a patient in a program of rehabilitation. His task is to learn to live with what he has left. He must accept the fact that growing older is a one-way and continuing process.

A moral emerges from the dilemma just propounded. Just being old takes up quite a bit of one's time. Just taking care of oneself requires a good deal of attention. But much of this health care does not require the services of highly trained practitioners.

Elder care problems lend themselves uniquely to solution by the patient—by self-medication. Who knows more about himself than the patient? Who is apt to give himself more tender and loving care? The problem becomes one of achieving professional supervision. The importance of self-care is now recognized in all the literature of progressive patient care.

From the standpoint of pure logic and basic economics, the greatest undeveloped resource in elder care is the patient himself. There is no conflict of interest. The patient has nothing more important to do. He will serve himself intelligently if he receives the advice and guidance of professional persons.

A practicing physician recently told this writer that the greatest opportunity to relieve the physician and nursing shortage in the United States was to delegate more duties and responsibilities to subordinate, paramedical personnel, which he defined to include the patient himself. He pointed out that we already condone the fact, while we decry the idea of self-medication. To illustrate this, he observed that many persons give themselves injections or other treatments for heart conditions, diabetes, and epilepsy.

Farewell to Medical Storehouses

This writer considers himself a crusader for the idea of keeping people out of institutions. Three decades ago, we worked hard to get people to enter hospitals. Later the physicians stressed early ambulation and short stays for hospital bed-patients. Now, the emphasis is rightly placed upon keeping people out of hospitals, even out of nursing homes, if possible. I do not want my fellow oldsters to become items of inventory—one-half being inmates and the other half caretakers of institutions.

What are the alternatives to institutional care? They are many, ranging from intermittent visits to comprehensive centers for ambulatory care to organized programs of personal companionship. Many chronically ill persons (most of them elderly) remain in general hospitals because there is no available alternative, such as a nursing home prepared to serve bed-fast patients. Likewise, many nursing homes assign bed facilities to ambulatory patients who might be equally well served through occasional visits by a physician, or nurse, or at a hospital.

The following substitutes for overnight incarceration are offered, singly or in combination. Each general hospital should offer a program of prevention, diagnosis, and treatment for ambulatory patients who are under the general supervision of a doctor, whether they are living in their own home, a foster home, an old folks home, or a nursing home.

Another alternative may be housekeeping assistance for one or two elderly persons who maintain their own establishment. Housekeeping services have been developed throughout the nation, especially in the cities, and they have contributed greatly to raising the self-respect and mental and physical health of the elderly.

Foster homes for the elderly have increased in recent years, usually as an aspect of social service and welfare, rather than as a health service. But the line need not be too sharply drawn. The important objective may be companionship and a sharing of interest and responsbility for daily needs and duties. Frequently, the host gains more than the guests from association during the long days and evenings.

The health care of an elderly person may require a degree of privacy not readily available in the household of the patient or relative. This dilemma could often be solved by the mere granting of money which would make it possible for the family to rent a house or apartment with an extra room for the elderly relative. Many social welfare regulations prohibit the granting of financial assistance for housing an elderly relative, even though the same agency would authorize the payment of four or five times as much to remove the patient unwillingly to an extended care facility. Hopefully, this penny-wise pound-foolish welfare policy will be revised as the institutions become too crowded to accept more inmates.

There is one type of elder care service which has not been fully developed, but which requires very little cash expenditure for its operation. This is the practice of *eldersitting*, by which individuals serve formally as temporary companions for each other, during an evening or an afternoon. The companions may be people of the same or different ages. Important matters are efficient management, and payment of the companions in cash, or in kind, for expenses incurred. Needless to say, such a program should include the practice of reciprocal visiting among the people registered as eldersitters.

There is great opportunity for public service in the establishment and operation of rehabilitation centers for elderly persons, which will emphasize activities of daily living. As mentioned previously, just being old takes up a lot of time, and the process ought to be undertaken with maximum possible efficiency. Such centers need not, of course, stress retraining for gainful employment, but they can demonstrate and teach methods of conserving energy in the business of self-care and self-support.

Such programs would naturally draw upon the competence of volunteer workers from among the elderly population, and would also constitute a wholesome form of occupational and or recreational therapy. This type of program is specially suitable for organization and encouragement by private philanthropy and nonofficial organizations. It may be the basis for experiment and research in the problems of voluntary and compulsory leisure.

Specialists in health have organized and encouraged informational and referral centers for people with chronic illness, including those who are merely aged and infirm. Needless to say, such programs are specially adapted to giving information and advice to those in need of occasional professional services, as well as persons who need continuous supervision and regularly provided professional care.

The Possibilities of Home Care

Home care programs have been frequently mentioned as desirable methods of caring for people with chronic illness, particularly those who are homebound, or find it difficult or impossible to travel, or be transported, to a central place for health service, such as a doctor's office, a hospital clinic, or a public health center. But home care is not new. People have been cared for in their homes for thousands of years. The new aspect is the bringing together of a variety of professional services, in the proper proportions, at the proper times, through an organization which coordinates the work of all health practitioners.

There is no single form of organization necessary to the establishment and operation of a good home care program. The home care may be limited or comprehensive. It may be continuous or intermittent. It may be interrelated with housekeeping or with recreation. The various Visiting Nurse Agencies have been engaging in home care for many years, and they constitute an important resource for any program, inasmuch as many of the duties are within the competence and understanding of the nursing profession.

The greatest drawback to the full development of home care service has been the relation between nurses and the private practitioners of medicine. As a general policy, home care must be initiated on the order and advice of a physician, who determines whether a patient needs a visiting nurse. A visiting nurse is not supposed to perform any professional services until authorized to do so by a licensed physician. The patient is expected to call a doctor to see if he needs a nurse. It would be more economical, and probably more effective, if he were expected to call a nurse to see if he needs a physician.

Elder care has many of the same economic characteristics as the practice of pediatrics. The individual patient is frequently not able to pay for the care he receives. The elderly patient is *no longer* in the labor force; the pediatric patient is *not yet* in the labor force. It is often said that a pediatrician spends much of his time treating parents rather than children. Likewise the geriatrist must become a specialist in family problems.

Some Events and Factors Leading to Medicare

The limited resources and the almost unlimited health care needs of elderly persons have been recognized for a long time by students of medical finance and administration. Most elderly persons are bad risks (moral hazards) from the standpoint of health insurance underwriting. To be sure, some individuals are self-supporting, self-reliant, and apparently healthy most of the time. But on the average, they will need medical care and advice more frequently than younger persons. An older person's demands may not always be justified from a scientific point of view, but the needs are nonetheless real to a person who is suffering mental or physical pain.

Voluntary health insurance plans have found that coverage for minor ailments, particularly among the elderly, are difficult to include in benefit programs. A few groups of physicians have worked successfully with this situation by judicious use of family doctors who are prepared to take as much time as necessary to understand the real or imagined illnesses of older patients.

When the Medicare program became part of the American scene, it became possible for physicians to spend greater amounts of time with older patients and to be reimbursed for their services. But Medicare is essentially a method of providing money for the payment of institutions and practitioners. It is not directly concerned with the efficiency of health production or the proper distribution of services to individuals in need of care.

Medicare as Miracle and Milestone

Federal Health Insurance Legislation effective July 1, 1966, suddenly changed the basis of financing much of the health service received by people over 65 years of age. During the first twelve months of operation, the Medicare program provided more than $2.5 billion for the payment of 5,000,000 hospital bills, and about $700 million for 10 million fees to physicians.

The calendar year 1967 showed a slight increase in hospital admissions. In addition, nearly 700,000 patients were admitted to extended-care facilities, more than 500,000 received outpatient care, and 300,000 were referred to home health programs. The total 1967 payments under the hospital insurance provisions were $2.9 billion.

Payments to physicians were slow in starting, but during 1967, the Social Security Administration reported that more than 24 million bills were received totalling $1.5 billion, of which about $1.1 billion was reimbursed under the program.

The sheer magnitude of these disbursements is of great significance. Within one year, they changed the national ratio of government expenditures from 25 to 35 percent of all health expenditures. They removed a substantial portion of the financial burden of sickness from nearly 20 million aged Americans. They materially affected the basis of current financing for many thousands of medical institutions and practitioners.

The Medicare program does not provide comprehensive health benefits. There are certain deductibles, co-insurance requirements, benefit exclusions, and dollar limitations. Among the exclusions are certain drugs, private nursing, dental care, physical examinations, eye tests and eyeglasses, and services to family members under 65 years of age. But the program is a giant step in the right direction. To change the metaphor, the national legislation has lifted the heaviest part of the load from the people least able to carry it. At the same time, it has guaranteed reimbursement to institutions and practitioners for services to many people whom they had previously served free, or at less than the cost of the care provided.

Not all Medicare reimbursement represents new money to finance health care for the American people. Some of the costs were previously met by patients' fees, insurance premiums, philanthropy, and other forms of state, local, and federal taxes. But the transfer of this financial load to the total population has laid the foundation for improvement in the quality and availability of health services.

Afterword: The Continuing Uncertainty

During the past five decades, the national bill for health care has increased astronomically, due to inflation, growth of population, and the provision of more and improved services for prevention, diagnosis, treatment, and rehabilitation. The vast majority of Americans are protected to some degree by private or public health insurance programs. Health care expenditures presently equal nearly 10 per cent of the gross national product.

These large increases in expenditure have not reduced public or private criticism regarding the burden of sickness costs. Why not? Because much health care financing has placed primary emphasis upon furnishing sick or disabled persons with money (or credit) instead of with the services essential to recovery. The additional money expenditures have often tended to assure the solvency of health care providers rather than delivery of necessary professional care.

An important development of the seventies has been the role played by Health Maintenance Organizations (HMOs). An HMO is a group practice–group payment program that provides health care benefits in terms of professional service rather than dollar amounts of cash (or credit). Some have been established as independent "group-health associations." Others are affiliated with or sponsored by Blue Cross or Blue Shield Plans, commercial insurance carriers, government agencies, industrial firms, medical societies, hospitals, or community nonprofit corporations.

Since the year 1972, the United States government has officially endorsed HMOs and made loans and grants to establish or expand programs in accord with specific administrative, economic and professional standards. There are now several hundred approved HMOs in the United States, with total enrollment of about 11,000,000 participants. The membership may be expected to reach 25 or 30 million within the next decade, according to Group Health Association of America in Washington, D.C., which serves as a coordinating body for group payment activities on a national basis.

Much criticism of health service proves, upon analysis, to be rebellion against the uncertain and unpredictable costs of health care. A health care provider (physician, hospital, dentist, nurse, or pharmacist) presents a patient with a bill for necessary services, and thereby becomes identified as the agency which caused the unplanned expenditure.

Practically everyone now approves of health insurance, at least in principle. The battle for health insurance is over, but the terms of peace are still under discussion. The general public deserves a comprehensive program of prevention, treatment, and rehabilitation, expressed in terms of services, not dollars.

The following question was asked of a large number of practicing physicians: "What do you think of the idea that physicians should receive regular full-time salaries for their professional advice?" A very large percentage gave exactly the same answer: "What salary did you have in mind?" And this reply was reasonable, for the main drawback to a salary may be its inadequacy. But certainly it would remove one incentive to provide services (even of high quality) which are unnecessary.

A health practitioner should be a producer, not merely a vendor, of professional service. The method and amount of reimbursement should motivate a policy of concern for a patient's health over and above concern for a practitioner's income. The piecework basis of payment seems unworthy of a professional who has special knowledge and skill obtained largely at public expense and financed largely by public contributions. The doctor is entitled to a guaranteed income based upon the value of his services throughout a period of time. He should be more interested in practicing medicine than selling it.

Several thousand persons heard my presentation in Constitution Hall, Washington, D.C., on April 24, 1934 at the fortieth national convention of the National League of Nursing Education, entitled "What Can the Public Do to Insure Good Nursing Service?" I called attention to the undefined roles of graduate, undergraduate, and practical nurses, and to professional relations with doctors of medicine. I startled the audience by questioning why it should be necessary to consult a physician to learn whether one needs a nurse. It seemed more logical to consult a nurse to learn whether one needs a doctor. Sooner or later, nursing responsibilities must be adjusted to the education and competence of nurses.

Development of nursing as a profession requires a clear definition of the role of the nurse in health care, which should be recognized by official agencies and other practitioners. Independence and authority to make decisions are criteria of all professions. Limits of responsibility for graduate nurses should be established by legislation, and educational programs should be adapted accordingly.

"Second" opinions are often established as a requirement for approval of surgery or other professional procedures, provided in accordance with health care insurance policies. Controversy has arisen over whose opinion should prevail. Should it be that of another surgeon, an internist, a general physician, a representative of a third-party payer? Obviously it should be someone with no financial interest in the fees which may be paid to the attending practitioner. Strictly speaking, the patient's opinion often becomes the deciding factor. He may receive conflicting opinions from members of the medical profession. In such cases, the patient decides whether he will have an operation, and who will perform the procedure. Second opinions might not reduce the total costs of medical care to a community or third-party payer. But they tend to raise professional standards by requiring careful consideration of many important professional services.

Co-insurance and deductible provisions are often used to limit the amount of care to which an insured person will be entitled. The purpose is declared to be the avoidance of unnecessary care, the conservation of providers' time and resources, and the containment of total costs to beneficiaries of a health care program. Undoubtedly co-insurance and deductibles accomplish these objectives. But their enforcement constitutes the control of medicine by arithmetic rather than professional judgment. The procedures are no boon to honest consumers, and are an implied insult to the integrity of ethical practitioners and responsible managers.

Legislators have shown great interest in programs which would provide payments to providers when the total costs reach catastrophic proportions that may exceed a person's total income or drive him into bankruptcy. Such instances face about one percent of the population annually. Care of catastrophic or terminal illness is a proper feature of a national or statewide program, but it should not precede or be substituted for the many services which are required in smaller amounts by more than half the population every year.

The United States Congress probably will not approve legislation for national comprehensive health care for the entire population during the next ten years. But there will be many changes in the organization and financing of health care during that period. Some will be continuations of trends already apparent.

An increasing number and proportion of physicians will practice their professions on an annual salary basis—good salaries, that is. The auspices will be private clinics, hospitals, industrial and commercial firms, governmental agencies, and health insurance organizations such as Blue Cross, Blue Shield, commercial carriers, and Health Maintenance Organizations.

Hospitals will become comprehensive health care centers with equal attention to vertical and horizontal patients. Outpatient visits will exceed the number of inpatient days at typical general hospitals, public or private.

Very few new hospitals will be established during the coming decade, except as parts of mergers and consolidations. Hospital size will be expressed in terms of volume and variety of services rather than floor space and bed capacity.

Official agencies will authorize and license various paramedical personnel to perform primary health care services, with specific responsibilities and privileges. Examples of such personnel are graduate nurses, rehabilitation therapists, trained midwives, and social work consultants.

Medical school clinical instruction will be provided in the private offices of practicing physicians, as well as in hospitals, nursing homes and patient residences.

Areawide planning agencies for comprehensive health care will be established throughout the country. Certificates of need will be required for all major changes or expansion of health care and facilities.

Medicare coverage for the elderly population will be revised to provide dentistry and prescription drugs. Medicaid programs for low-income groups will be merged with Medicare.

Health care insurance benefits will be expressed in terms of professional services, not cash allowances. Malingering will be controlled by authoritative professional judgment rather than deductible or co-insurance provisions.

Hospitals will be increasingly staffed by full-time or contractual attending physicians. This trend will occur in governmental, nonprofit, and investor-owned institutions.

Special-duty nursing service in hospitals will be provided by the institutions' professional staff on an hourly or fee-for-service basis.

Interest, depreciation, and capital replacement allowances will be included in reimbursement formulas for health care. But these allowances will be placed in separate funds to be expended in accord with certified community needs.

Supervised self-care will be developed under professional guidance, in the interest of more effective use of health care knowledge and skill.

Group practice in health care enables each specialist to serve alternately as teacher and student. The whole is greater than the sum of the parts.

Group payment applies the law of averages to control the ravages of sickness and disability, and to place health care in the family budget with other necessities.

Health care facilities have been provided by the general public in the interest of service to individuals. They should be planned and utilized to furnish the greatest good for the greatest number.

An individual patient can be trusted, under supervision, to give himself tender and loving health care. He has no conflict of interest, and nothing more important to do.

Appendix A:
Chronological List of Books and Brochures
by C. Rufus Rorem (1928–1970)

Date of Publication	Title and Publisher
June 1928	*Accounting Method* (textbook), University of Chicago Press (UCP)
November 1930	*The Public's Investment in Hospitals*, UCP
January 1931	*Private Group Clinics*, UCP; reprinted 1970 by Milbank Memorial Fund
July 1931	*The Municipal Doctor System in Rural Saskatchewan*, UCP
July 1931	*The Middle-Rate Plan at Massachusetts General Hospital*, Julius Rosenwald Fund (JRF)
January 1932	*Annual Medical Service in Private Clinics*, JRF
April 1932	*The Costs of Medicines*, with R. P. Fischelis, UCP
July 1932	*Second Year of the Middle-Rate Plan*, with Clyde Frost, M.D., and Elizabeth Day, JRF
September 1932	*The Crisis in Hospital Finance*, with Michael M. Davis, UCP
December 1932	*Group Payment for Medical Care at Standard Oil Company of Louisiana*, with John H. Musser, M.D., JRF
January 1933	*The Costs of Medical Care*, with I. S. Falk and M. D. Ring, UCP
October 1935	*Hospital Accounting and Statistics*, American Hospital Association (AHA)
June 1936	*Quality of Medical Care at a Midwestern Private Clinic*, with John H. Musser, M.D., JRF

January 1940	*Non-Profit Hospital Service Plans,* AHA
March 1944	*Blue Cross Hospital Service Plans,* (AHA)
April 1946	*Verbatim Testimony before United States Senate Committee on Education and Labor,* reprinted by AHA
March 1949	*Physicians' Private Offices at Hospitals,* AHA Monograph No. 5
April 1963	*Satellite Hospitals,* with P. B. Hallen, United States Public Health Service, HM00184
September 1964	*Guide and Procedures for Long Range Planning,* Hospital Review and Planning Council of Southern New York, HRP
June 1968	*Capital Financing for Hospitals,* HRP
March 1970	*Economics of Medical Care,* chapter IV of *Depth and Extent of the Geriatric Problem,* Charles C. Thomas, Inc.

Appendix B:
Articles by C. Rufus Rorem Published in Journals and Magazines (1925–1971)

(Listed chronologically by publication or publisher; does not includ·
articles reprinted in this volume)

Accounting Review

March 1927	Similarities of Accounting and Statistics
September 1928	Social Control through Accounts
December 1928	Differential Costs
June 1930	Cost Analysis for Hospitals
March 1932	The Costs of Medical Care
June 1936	Uniform Hospital Accounting
June 1937	Accounting Theory: A Critique
September 1937	Replacement Cost in Accounting Valuation

American Academy for the Advancement of Science, Bulletin

March 1936	Recent Developments in Group Hospitalization
1939, Vol. 9	pp. 219–23 Mental Health and Medical Economics

American College of Surgeons, Bulletin

April 1938	Influence of Insurance on Health Service
June 1939	Trends in Hospital Care Insurance

American Economic Security, Chamber of Commerce of U.S.

January 1944	Community Hospital and Medical Plans
June 1952	Can Hospital Costs Be Controlled?

American Hospital Association, Bulletin

November 1933	Hospital Care in the Family Budget
May 1934	Policies and Procedures of Group Hospitalization
September 1934	Group Budgeting for Hospital Care
January 1935	Group Budgeting for Hospital Care
April 1935	Progress in Group Hospitalization

American Hospital Association, Transactions

September 1931	Cost Analysis—An Aid to Financing
September 1932	Bed Occupancy in General Hospitals
September 1933	What the Periodic Payment Plan Has Demonstrated
September 1934	Group Hospitalization, Report and Round Table
September 1934	Group Hospitalization—A Formal Paper
October 1935	Group Hospitalization Report
September 1936	Group Hospitalization Report
September 1937	Recent Developments in Hospital Care Insurance
September 1938	How to Start a Plan

American Journal of Public Health

January 1949	Rising Costs and Group Payment
July 1958	Physicians' Private Offices at Hospitals
August 1958	Developments in Group Practice
March 1964	Community Hospital Planning Associations

American Medical Association, Journal

January 11, 1930	Control and Types of Hospital Service in the U.S.
January 18, 1930	Hospital Facilities and Capital Investment in the U.S.
June 11, 1932	Percentage of Occupancy in American Hospitals

Blue Cross Association, Bulletin

April 1959	Hospital Care a Community Affair
May 1960	Justin Ford Kimball Award Address

Canadian Hospital Journal

September 1932	Cost of Medical Care

Canadian Medical Journal

Autumn 1954	Economics of Group Practice

Druggist, the

March 1932	Service of Pharmacy in Medical Care

Duke University Law Journal

Autumn 1938	Legislation for Hospital Service Plans (with M. J. Norby)

Encyclopaedia Britannica

1957	Accounting—Official Entry
1963	Hospital—Official Entry
1971	Hospital—Official Entry

Friends Journal (Book Reviews)

July 1965	*Freedom's Advocate,* Levenstein and Agar
January 1966	*D-Days and Dayton,* J.R. Tompkins
August 1966	*Riots, U.S.A. (from 1765 to 1965),* Willard A. Heaps
June 1967	*A Fellowship of Discontent,* Hans J. Hillebrand
October 1967	*The Enlightenment (Rise of Modern Paganism),* Peter Gay
February 1968	*The Future as Nightmare,* Mark R. Hillegas
February 1969	*Beyond Economics,* Kenneth E. Boulding

Georgia Hospital Association Bulletin

December 1959	Associations and Professional Growth

Hospital Financial Management

June 1954	Patients Get a Bargain for Their Hospital Dollar
May 1955	Horizons for Accounting
June 1962	Prologue and Prophecy in Hospital Accounting
September 1963	Accounting and Community Planning
July 1972	Prologue and Prophecy (Ten Years After)

Hospital Management

June 1931	Hospital Endowment
April 1957	Hospital Costs
June 1965	Nursing as a Profession

Hospital Progress

February 1931	Capital Expenditures in Hospitals
August 1954	Purchasing Functions
March 1964	Operation of a Hospital Planning Association

Hospitals (Journal of the American Hospital Association)

April 1936	Hospitalization Plans Forge Ahead
January 1937	Program on Group Hospitalization
May 1938	Approved List of Hospital Care Plans
November 1938	Outline for Program of Approved Plans
January 1940	Non-Profit Hospitals

March 1940	Developments in Hospital Service Plans
January 1946	Truman's Health Program
February 1948	Joint Purchasing in Philadelphia
March 1950	Group Purchasing
January 1953	Impact of Third Party Payments
May 1953	The Case of Mr. X, a "Free" Patient
August 1956	Physicians' Offices at Hospitals
March 1957	Rising Costs
March 1964	Objectives and Criteria for Hospital Planning

Hospital Tidings (Hahnemann Hospital)

Autumn 1952	Nursing of the Future

Hospital World

December 1961	Quality of Care (an Interview)

Journal of Accountancy

July 1929	Accounting as a Science
October 1950	Hospital Accounting (Cost Analysis)

Journal of Business

January 1929	Accounting (Esquerre)—Book Review
July 1929	Business Value (Summary of Doctoral Thesis)

Journal of Medical Education

January 1965	Public Policy and Financing for Health Services (with Robert M. Sigmond)

Journal of Political Economy (Book Reviews)

June 1926	*Trends in Swedish Economics,* Bertil Ohlin
October 1925	*Accounting Principles of Federal Income Tax,* Kohler
May 1926	*Accounting for General Contractors,* Grant
August 1927	*Survey Course in Accounting,* McCarty and Amidon
December 1927	*Principles of Accounting,* Kohler and Morrison
June 1928	*The General Accounting Office,* Darrell Smith

Kiwanis Magazine

September 1934	Hospital Care in the Family Budget
September 1938	Hospital Care Insurance

Literary Digest

May 16, 1931	How Canada Keeps Its Doctors

Medical Care

April 1941   Non-Profit Hospital Service Plans

Medical Economics

November 1932   Do Physicians Want Contract Practice?
March 1934   Middlemen Not Allowed

Minnesota Medicine

October 1937   Health Problems from Lay Viewpoints

Modern Hospital

January 1931   What Is Part Pay Service?
July 1931   Group Clinics: Where, How and Whom They Serve
May 1933   California Gets Under Way
January 1934   Group Hospitalization for Goodyear Employees
July 1935   In a Small Hospital Uniform Accounting Is Helpful
August 1938   Hospital Care: Service, Not Cash
August 1947   Economics of Hospital Charges
December 1947   Contract Rates
February 1949   Practical Nurse Training in Philadelphia
December 1950   "No Color Line" But No Alternative
September 1951   We Can't Afford Cut Rate Accounting
October 1951   We Can't Afford Cut Rate Accounting, continued
January 1952   Factors That Influence Free Service
July 1953   Commercial Insurance
August 1946   Job of a Hospital Council
March 1957   Physicians' Private Offices at Hospitals
March 1962   Twenty Questions for Hospital Planning

National League for Nursing, Proceedings

April 1934   What Can the Public Do to Insure Good Nursing
                        Service?

Nursing, American Journal of

April 1933   Is Student Nursing an Economy?
June 1935   Health Insurance, What, Why and Where?
July 1935   Hospital Care in the Family Budget
February 1937   Group Hospitalization
July 1941   Nurses and Hospital Service Plans

Radio (National Advisory Radio Council on Education)

December 1934   Doctors, Dollars and Disease

Rhode Island Hospital Association Bulletin

March 1946	Rhode Island Leads the Way

Southern Hospitals

January, 1952	Survival by Cooperation
December, 1953	Patients Get a Bargain for Their Hospital Dollar

State Government

May 1939	Voluntary Hospital Care Insurance

Survey Graphic

January 1930	Private Group Clinics
March 1935	Hospital Care in the Family Budget

Trustee

July 1951	Systematic Accounting
April 1954	Planning Standards: Evidence of Community Need
May 1954	Planning Standards: Prospects of High Utilization
June 1954	Planning Standards: Assurance of Adequate Financing
July 1954	Planning Standards: Accordance with Professional Trends
January 1958	Quality and Financing of Hospital Care

Viewpoints (Health Insurance)

December 1967	Relating Planning to Health Service Problems

Western Hospital Review

March 1933	Guiding Principles for Group Hospitalization
November 1933	Nursing: An Economic Paradox

World Hospitals (formerly Nosokomeion)

March 1932	Some Hospital Financial Problems
September 1936	Hospitals as Social Capital
August 1937	Uniform Hospital Accounting
April 1969	Progressive Patient Care

Yankton College Bulletin

June 1935	Frontiers of Intelligence (Commencement Address)

About the Author

1894—Born Radcliffe, Iowa. Diploma Mason City, Ia. H.S. 1911
1916—A.B. Oberlin College, with honors in Political Science and election to
    Phi Beta Kappa
1923—Certified Public Accountant, State of Indiana
1925—A.M. Commerce and Administration, University of Chicago
1929—Ph.D. Commerce and Administration, University of Chicago
1935—LL.D. Yankton College

1916–17, 1919–22—Goodyear Tire and Rubber Company
1917–18—U.S. Military Service
1922–24—Assistant Professor of Economics and Dean of Men, Earlham
    College
1924–29—Instructor to Associate Professor of Accounting, Assistant Dean,
    School of Business, University of Chicago
1929–31—Economist and Accountant, Committee on the Costs of Medical
    Care, Washington, D.C.
1931–36—Associate for Medical Services, Julius Rosenwald Fund, Chicago.
1937–46—Director, Blue Cross Commission, American Hospital Association,
    Chicago
1947–59—Executive Director, Hospital Council of Philadelphia
1960–64—Executive Director, Hospital Planning Association of Allegheny
    County, Pittsburgh
1964–69—Special Consultant, Health and Hospital Planning Council of
    Southern New York, New York City
1969–74—Special Consultant, Blue Cross Association (Chicago)

Awards
1960—Justin Ford Kimball, American Hospital Association
1969—Distinguished Service, American Association for Hospital Planning
1972—Trustee Award, Hospital Financial Management Association
1977—Honorary Membership, American Institute of Certified Public
    Accountants
1979—Prepayment Pioneer, 50th Anniversary, Blue Cross and Blue Shield
    Associations
1980—Distinguished Service, Hospital Association of Pennsylvania

* * * * * * * * * * * * * * *

Life Member of American Hospital Association and American Public
Health Association